There is quite a bit of Potteries dialec
which I have added a translation at the b;

My thanks go to Pat and Mel, who I know from the Werrington table tennis club, for their help in checking over the Potteries dialect and to Pat for proofreading the manuscript.

My thanks also go to Mark Brereton for giving me the initial idea for this book, after telling me numerous ghost stories that are associated with Ash Hall and the surrounding area.

My thanks also go to Mervyn Edwards for his continuous promotion of "Footsteps in the Past", to which this book is a sequel.

© 2019 Margaret Moxom. All rights reserved

No part of this book may be reproduced, stored in a retrieval system or transmitted by any means without the written permission of the author.

The views expressed in this work are solely those of the author.

Front and back covers paintings are produced by the author

FOOTSTEPS IN THE PAST

THE SECRET

CONTENTS
CHAPTER 1 – The Warning 1

CHAPTER 2 – The Aftermath 22

CHAPTER 3 – The Reform Bill 49

CHAPTER 4 – School 62

CHAPTER 5 – Werrington 78

CHAPTER 6 – Bucknall 88

CHAPTER 7 – The Visit 111

CHAPTER 8 – Geoffrey 118

CHAPTER 9 - Coming of the Railway 129

CHAPTER 10 – The Train Ride 137

CHAPTER 11 – Cellarhead 158

CHAPTER 12 – Job Meigh Estate 164

CHAPTER 13 – North Staffordshire Royal Infirmary 177

CHAPTER 15 – The workhouse Infirmary 201

CHAPTER 15 – Spectres 217

CHAPTER 16 – St Mary's Church 226

CHAPTER 17 – Change has Come 242

CHAPTER 18 – The Secret Revealed 258

CHAPTER 19 – The Inquest 267

CHAPTER 20 – House of Commons Report 283

Translation 287
Acknowledement 314

CHAPTER 1 – THE WARNING

I was just doing my rounds, as community nurse, on the morning of Tuesday, 3rd May 1881. I'd been over to visit one of my patients in Brookhouse Lane, over the back of the Ash Hall, which had been built by Job Meigh, just before the Pottery riots of 1842. Job Meigh had been one of the entrepreneur potters in the Potteries of Stoke-on-Trent. He had made his fortune in this industry, having bought all the land and farms hereabouts and had built additional properties, during the time that I'd known him, thus adding to his empire. My John had worked for him all this time, on his building and maintenance projects, as well as being gardener and handyman at Ash Hall, having originally worked at Job Meigh's pottery, in what is now the Meigh Lane car park in Hanley. I call him "my John" but we'd actually separated some time ago. John continued to live at the gatehouse at the rear of Ash Hall, in Brookhouse Road, while I had taken one of the old stone cottages in the old village of Washerwall.

I was taking a footpath through the moorlands from Brookhouse Lane, to get onto the Bridle Path, then on to see a patient at one of the farms. I was in a bit of a daydream, I suppose, not really paying attention to my surroundings, just taking care of my footing as the path was unmade and overgrown. I was coming up to the little wooden bridge that went over a brook. The area was overgrown with a copse of trees, which deeply shaded the path and cut out the sunshine.

All of a sudden I heard a voice and looked up. What I saw was a filmy sort of bright white light directly ahead of me. The light was hovering slightly above the path.

"Who's there?" I called out, shielding my eyes from the glare. "If you want to rob me, I've no money on me." The area was known for miscreants, out for easy money from unsuspecting travellers, not forgetting the number of Irish who had infiltrated Stoke, following the Irish famine. The Irish weren't especially menacing, just begging for food, or harassing you for any work that might be going, but there was also a drunken element, be they Irish or local, who were out for a fight and to steal anything they could get their hands on. It wasn't a place to be at night time. But this wasn't night time and any drunks would probably still be recovering before taking to the booze once again.

I called out again, "Who's there?" as I watched intensely this hovering bright light edged closer to me. My heart was beginning to race now. Should I run back, go round another way? And, if I did, would whoever, whatever it was, follow me?

I then heard a voice, a female voice, calling softly, "Jane, Jane."

– that was my name, so this person knew me!

"Who are you ….do I know you?" I replied, my voice trembling slightly, showing a bit of the fear I was beginning to feel.

"Yes... you know me........I am Jane." came the reply. The misty light then descended onto the path and began to form the outline of a figure. This 'Jane' was softly silhouetted in the hazy light and seemed to be wearing dark trousers and a blouse, the type worn by nurses. I was astonished as much by the clothes the figure wore as the figure itself. I hadn't seen a woman wearing trousers ...... at least not for about 40 years.... That's when it began slowly to dawn on me..... 40 years, what was I doing 40 years ago? I'd got so accustomed to my way of life, set in my routine, that the past had disappeared into a vague memory. Was my memory playing tricks with me – and why should I remember seeing women in trousers? – No women wore trousers – it just wasn't done.

As the haziness cleared I could see a pleasant-looking girl of about 25 years, with long fair hair. Then, I almost swooned and I grabbed hold of the nearest tree to save myself from falling. My hand went to my mouth to stifle a scream.

"Don't be afraid, Jane." came from the apparition."Don't you recognise me?"

"Y..es" I stuttered. "You....you're ....me!"

"Yes, Jane....... I died here in 2019, in Bridle Path. We, as one entity, found ourselves sent back to 1842 to discover the secret of John's death. We were then one person, but our paths split somehow. You stayed in the 19th century to remain with John. We could not both be alive. I was the one to die. You changed history by staying with John and John didn't die."

"Yes, I remember. I didn't know the consequences at the time of wanting to stay with John. I'm sorry it had to come to that".... I continued, still rather taken aback and frightened. I'd been in the 19th century now for 39 years – I was 64 in this day and age. Was she coming to return me to the 21st century or had I died this moment, now, in Bridle Path and she was coming to join us together in some way, to bring the circle to a close. I couldn't think straight but managed to get out, "What do you wish from me? Why are you here?"

"I have a warning for you, Jane. Your son, Alfred, is in danger. You must go to him."

"Alfred, oh Alfred. He's at the Lillydale Colliery, what's happened?"

"You must go to him" was all the apparition said and then started to fade and gradually disappeared.

The bright light had gone, leaving the copse in darkness again.

I was in such distress. "Oh God, Alfred" I called out. Something terrible had happened, or was about to. I finally got my wits together and started running back along the path and onto the road for Washerwall. Getting there, very much out of breath, I shouted out down the little lane that there was danger at Lillydale Colliery.

People came out of their houses and, seeing my distress, Mr Bowyer offered to hitch up his pony and cart to take me and anyone else who could help, to the colliery.

We shouted out on the way to people in the streets, as the horse and cart raced down Ash Bank to Ruxley Road, on the left, to get to the colliery. I didn't know what else to do, wringing my hands and very tearful. I saw John along the way. He was working at one of the farms and called to him.

I could see the heaps of spoil on the horizon, as we turned left into Ubberley Road, in the direction of Ubberley Hall. There was no quicker way of getting there as there was no other crossing over the river, which ran from the moors and flowed past to the north of the pit.

On getting there, John made a dash for the entrance to the pit and descended with quite a few others. It seems there'd been an explosion and the miners were trapped.

Then I overheard one chap shouting out that the water had been tapped and was rushing into the thirling. I think he must have been the new manager, Enoch Perrins. He was calling out for help, for people to go down and try to rescue as many as they could. Just at that moment there was a cracking "boom", the most dreadful of all sounds in a mining village, the unmistakable crack of an explosive blast. It seemed that the force of the air current had disturbed some gas hanging about to be driven into the naked flames of the candles, and the whole place had exploded. Everyone began screaming and sobbing around me, frantic anxiety depicted on everyone's face. Smoke, soot and dust, peppered with sparks, were now spiralling upward from the chimney fan to form a black and acrid canopy over the stricken pit.

Something of Enoch Perrins' thoughts and emotions must have shone in his face when his eyes met those of wives and mothers, whose menfolk were still in the pit. Whatever were his failings, he never wished to see his mine disintegrate into rubble, with loss of life. I wasn't sure he was a capable man, having managed the mine for such a short time but his job now was to contact the hospitals and police and local collieries. Contact with survivors, if any, must be achieved at all costs.

Within half an hour only, the water had risen so rapidly it had filled most of the workings.

Several volunteers and men from neighbouring collieries, at great personal risk of their own lives, had ventured down. One by one miners were brought out. Thomas Plant, Anthony Barlow and William Tabbinor were saved from drowning.

I went over to help and was down on my knees, tending to as many as I could. Dr Knight was there too. It seemed that they'd only noticed William Tabbinor, as they'd seen his hand moving above the water and heard gurgling sounds – they'd only just saved him as he was within seconds of drowning. It was only with great difficulty that they got him out. George Phillips was found near the edge of the water, just in time to be saved. He was unconscious from the effects of the after damp. A number of fathers and mothers broke the cordon and were rushing towards the volunteers bringing the men out. A number of them were groaning and weeping hysterically, others turned away with heads bowed after finding their family member hadn't been brought out. Stretchers were brought forward and Thomas Plant, Anthony Barlow and George Philipps were taken over to the North Staffs Infirmary.

A dead body was then brought out. I could do nothing for him. He was recognised by his screaming wife as Edward Clewlow.

I recalled Alfred having told me that this wasn't an extensive colliery and not very lucrative as it had changed hands many times. It had been opened about 25 years previously by Mr Forrester, Mr Gerrard and Mr Hawkes. Mr Enoch Perrins was the present proprietor but had only owned it for less than a year. Only 16 men were engaged in the pit, working with just a candle attached to their helmets, for light. Some of them had been driving a thirling, or connecting tunnel, on the north side of the south dip at a depth of about 160 yards. It was anticipated that there might be a possible influx of water from an old working and two bore holes nine feet long and an inch in diameter had been kept ahead all through the driving as a precautionary measure. Obviously this precautionary measure wasn't enough. My Alfred was the fireman on site.

I don't know how long I was there but realised, when I saw the rescuers, coughing and spluttering, smeared with coal dust and soaking wet, exiting from the mine with no other bodies, that there had been no sign of Alfred or John. The rescue had been called off as the water was too high. The weary men, sat down to rest and to empty their water bottles into their burning gullets. Mr Perrins sat apart, his head cupped between his hands.

Maybe Alfred had been at the coal face and no-one could get to him. The ridiculous hope, that I was desperately clinging onto was that he'd found a pocket of air and would be rescued later. I found myself screaming, "John" over and over. I was trembling and moaning....Then a shout came from the pit head, calling for me. "Way've got John. 'E's in a bad way." I ran over. "Way dragged 'im ite o' watter, 'es near drowneded." I fell to my knees over him and started performing CPR, something the locals had never seen before and were looking on in astonishment. He had no pulse. Then, water started dribbling out of his mouth and he started coughing and spluttering. He'd virtually drowned in the pit, trying desperately to get to keep his head above water and get to a place where he could find air. With the CPR, John spewed out the water he had taking into his lungs. He'd been dragged out by the other rescuers, who had been desperately searching, like John, for any trapped colliers who had survived the explosion. He was alive – covered with coal dust and burns to his face and hands. "Oh John, thank goodness" I shouted to him. I'd been there helping these wretched fathers, husbands and sons but, when John was brought out, he was all I cared about and rushed to him. He began to come to. I managed to grab hold of a spare blanket to wrap round him, but as he was trying to get up, he suddenly cried out in pain and grabbed his chest, then fell back again.

I realised he had had a heart attack. He was 70 – he should never have gone down there, but he wasn't thinking of his own life – he was trying to save our son. There was no pulse so I started CPR on him again Finally, after what seemed an eternity, I got a pulse. I started screaming out for someone to get him back to the cottage where I lived and a couple of lads finally came back with a door they'd wrenched off its hinges and loaded John onto it. I wanted him back at the cottage so I could look after him myself. As they were carrying him to the horse-drawn cart, I'd came in, he murmured something and I bent down to hear, "Ah codna fayned 'im. Ah trayed."

"I know you did, John, you tried your best." I answered, but John's eyes had glazed over and his head fell to one side. I felt his pulse again – there was nothing. "Put him down, quick." I shouted to the two men. "He's not breathing, he's having another heart attack". I started on the CPR again. "Come on John, breathe." I was shouting at him, between compressions and breaths, whispering the numbers of compressions before giving two breaths, checking his pulse and continuing with the compressions. It was exhausting work, down on my knees, but I wasn't going to give up. "Don't die John, please don't die."

At last, to my relief, I felt a pulse, "Right, lads, pick him up, take him to the cart, be very careful with him please."

So, here we were back at the cottage. We couldn't get John up the narrow stairs to the bedroom, so I asked the lads to bring a single bed down and place it in the living room. It was a bit of a task, pushing and shoving and, while they did that, I gave John an injection of morphine. Dr Knight prescribed me supplies of this regularly to use to help my very sick and dying patients. Then I cleared a place for the bed, moving the table over. I asked the lads to keep John on the door, with both placed on the bed. I gave him an injection of morphine. I then took off John's wet clothes and boots and put a night gown on him. I'd cleaned him up as best as possible and applied salve to the burns on his face and hands and bandaged him - luckily they weren't deep burns, as, ironically, the water from the flooded pit would have helped. I'd also rolled him over so I could put a blanket and sheet over the door and had covered him up. I knew that, if he had another heart attack, he needed to be on something hard, otherwise I'd have to drag him onto the floor, to perform CPR again, which I wouldn't be able to do. There were no CPR paddles in those days, not even any electricity. Oh I wish I could miracle up something from the future and bring it here. An Adrenalin injection maybe, but that didn't exist either.

I'd stay there, by his side, keeping an eye on him for any response, either positive or negative, checking his pulse regularly. That's all I could do. I felt so helpless. If I could only transport myself into the future, I could bring back a defibrillator or even Aspirin, again something which hadn't been discovered yet. Laudanum, a mixture of opium and alcohol (a highly addictive narcotic drug), was super cheap and could easily be purchased from a local chemist! Laudanum was often used to ease pain on the deathbed and for a wide range of ailments and diseases, such as cholera, menstrual cramps, common colds, yellow fever and dysentery, but with so many side-effects, so I wasn't going to use Laudanum on John. Morphine was addictive too, but more effective. I didn't want to use too much on my John. I would just have to wait and see how he responded.

I sat by his side, looking at him while he slept. He looked so peaceful now that the drug had eased his pain, but so pale. I looked at his face and I cried to see it so close to me. The years had taken their toll, but so had they on me. They were hard times. His hair was no longer fair and wavy. The fair hair had been replaced by grey, and some of the curl had gone, but he still had a full head of hair and his body, in general, still showed muscle tone. There were areas where the skin had formed into small folds, like the tide going out in the sand. I had these myself, at the tops of my arms and legs. There were deeply etched lines around his eyes, which were closed, so I couldn't see his beautiful blue eyes; the skin and muscle tone around his throat showed his age, plus I could discern a ruddy sheen to his face, showing through the pallor that the heart attack had brought on. Of course, the ruddy colour would be through being out in all weathers, outside most of the time, building new houses and doing repair work. The wind would have drawn those lines but, to me, he was still handsome.

I thought of all the years gone by. I thought of how much loss there had been - so much loss, and sorrow. At first we had been happy, on the whole - swings and roundabouts as with every marriage but, whatever trials and tribulations we had gone through, we'd been there for each other. But that was at first. I was now 64 and John was 70. He should never have gone into that pit at his age, but our son was down there. Mines employed all ages, male and female, and kids from seven years old to men of 70 were working down there. Although women weren't allowed underground anymore, they had been, hauling and pushing the truck loads of coal. They were a tough lot these miners.

I sat myself in the rocking chair beside the bed and started to cry. I didn't know whether Alfred had been brought out alive or not, but I had to be with John.

My head was in a turmoil and, all of a sudden, the room started to spin – everything around me seemed to change. I was in water, a deep, ocean. Everything was black, deep dark, eerie black with no possibility of seeing land. I was paddling water, floating, my skirt billowing out around me. I was cold, freezing, wet. I shouted out but my voice just echoed around me. I was so frightened I started to scream. Screaming, screaming..... but nothing.... Just my own screams echoing over and over, getting louder and louder. I held my hands over my ears to try stop the sounds. I was shivering to my bones, all hope had gone. The water was lapping over me and I was swallowing water. I'd surely drown. This was the end – I was going to die..... But, all of a sudden I felt something touch me – seaweed – what was it – a fish – a shark even, but it was warm. I reached out and touched it. It was a hand, a human hand. It was warm, so not dead. I reached out to the form attached to that hand and drew myself closer, feeling that body. It was John. He was alive and breathing, but not aware.... asleep maybe. I tried to wake him but had no response. He was just floating there, with me.... But, it was a relief somewhat and my panic eased slightly. At least I wasn't alone. I had to try to keep him afloat.

The room went back to normal. I was stunned, deep shock was setting in. I was still shaking. I attempted to take deep breaths to try to slow down my pulse rate and calm my terror. After a few minutes, my mind cleared and I began to understand that this must have been an hallucination relating to our poor son deep in the pit, up to his neck in water. It was so awful, I had to try to keep this out of my mind, otherwise I could see myself breaking down and be no use to anyone. I got up and made myself a cup of tea, with sugar – I don't normally take sugar, but I thought it might help - and went back to the chair beside John.

I started to doze and found myself dreaming, thankfully not of the deep inky-black water, although I was sure this image would haunt me and not be very far from my thoughts. It was bound to remain there, hovering, until Alfred was safe, or his body was found.

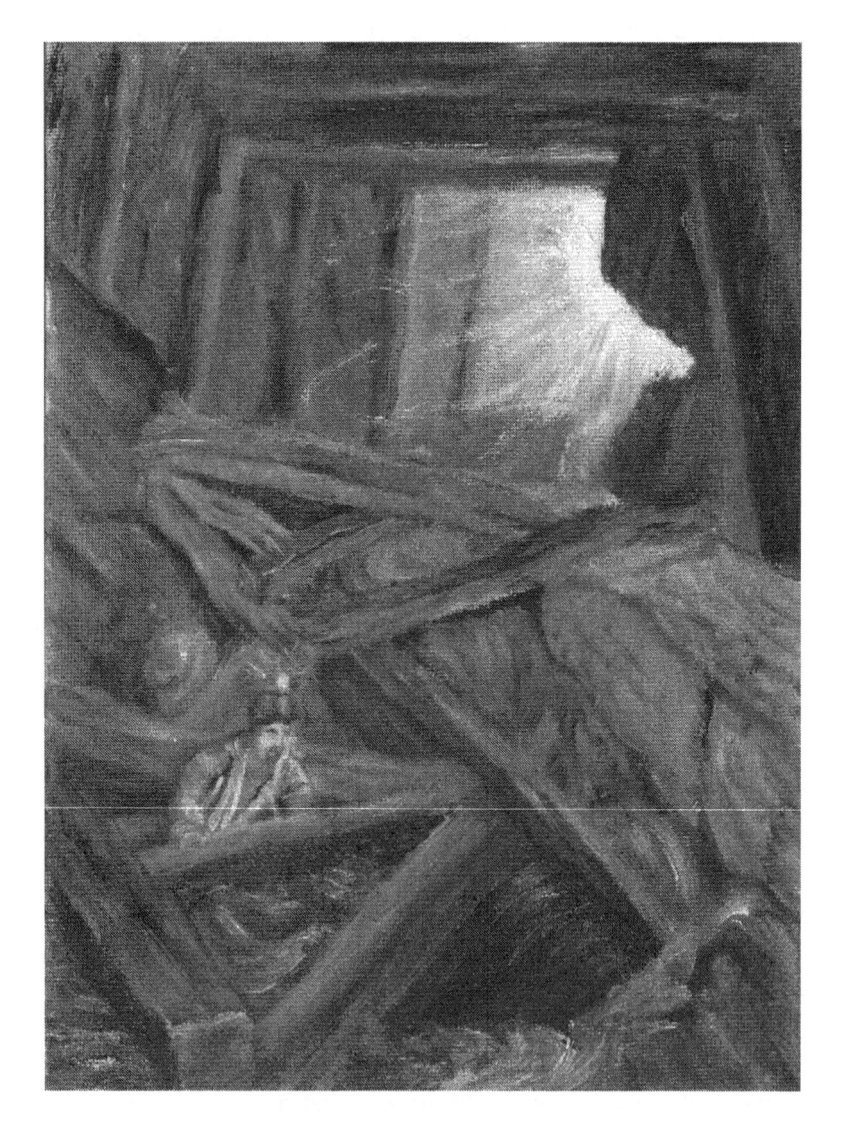

(Dream)

I woke up and looked around. I was in one of the bedrooms at the Ash Hall. It was 1842. I felt terribly weak still and my head was spinning with all that had happened in the last few days. The shock of finding myself in the midst of the Pottery Riots of 1842 and wondering whether I'd ever get out alive, was still so prominent in my memory and I found myself trembling, wanting to cry. John and I had been hiding behind the wall at the Big House in Burslem while thousands of marauding, violent, starving potters and miners stood up against the army at the top of Moorlands Avenue in Burslem. Captain Powys, on his charger with his sword held high, was reading out the Riot Act to them, telling the populace to go home quietly, in the name of Queen Victoria. The crowd retaliated, shouting out that they had nothing to go home to and they wanted food. They were carrying stones and sticks and whatever they had found to defend themselves with or to attack anyone who came up against them, even the army with their rifles raised against them. It was a stand-off. Then one of the soldiers saw a lad, Josiah Heapy, bend to pick up a stone, as if to throw at them, and turned his rifle round, aimed and shot him in the head. That shot reverberated all around. Josiah's blood splattered against the wall, behind which we were hiding. I had buried my head in John's chest to stifle a scream and John was holding me tight. Any slight whiff by the army that there was someone behind that wall and we would have been dead meat.

On hearing the shot and seeing Josiah's head blown to pieces, there was a deadly silence in the crowd for a second, to be replaced by murmurings, then all of a sudden the crowd took flight, running in all directions, for their lives. More shots rang out, aimed mainly above the heads of the starving masses but some of the army followed swinging their swords menacingly at whoever got in their way. People were falling over themselves to escape, tripping over the wounded, in their bid to flee the devils on horseback.

John and I waited until the crowds and army had passed. The soldiers were driving the masses along, whilst the special constables were placed opposite every avenue to the market place to prevent a fresh rush of people. We had managed to get ourselves to the back of the Shambles, but kept well back, not to be entangled in the crowd and finally managed to get on the road back to Ash Hall.

I was shattered. We'd been on the go since early morning, with no sustenance of any kind and we'd walked for miles, in the summer heat. I just couldn't go another step, feeling sick to the bone as we approached Ash Hall, only to find that some of the crowd had made their way to Ash Hall and were berating Job Meigh, threatening to set fire to the hall. Job Meigh was standing on the steps at the entrance, attempting to appease the crowd. I don't remember much more. I think I must have passed out.

The next thing I remember is waking up here with John, Job Meigh, Dinah the cook, and a doctor, looking at me with very worried expressions. John was calling me his wife to be. Yes...., I remember now. I'd said I'd loved him and never wanted to leave him and John had proposed. Then everything went dizzy again and I felt myself drifting away. John was holding on tight, begging me not to leave him. It was a horrible feeling. I was dying......., but I wasn't dying in that bed, I was dying in the Bridle Path that runs alongside the estate and I had been shouting out, over and over again, "Let me stay, I don't want to go back."

"Oh God, what have I done", I shouted out - but there was no-one to hear- as the full weight of the reality of what I had begged for gradually engulfed me, in a stranglehold. I had begged to stay with John in the 19th century and my prayers had been answered, but this meant. I could never go back to the 21st century. My 21st century persona had died in Bridle Path.

Just then Dinah Chetwynd, Job Meigh's cook, entered the room. "'ere ducky, ah've bought yer a nice cuppa tay. Ah 'heard yer calling, so thought yer must be awake. 'ow are yer feeling?"

"Thank you Dinah. Just what I need. Yes, I'm awake but not feeling 100%. I'm a bit confused. I've no idea how I got here or what happened. All I remember is collapsing in Bridle Path, and there was a crowd of people confronting Mr Meigh on the steps. Although I vaguely remember that John was here and, - tell me if I'm wrong or have made this up in my fuddled mind, - but did John propose to me and did I accept?"

"Yes, ducky. That indeed did 'appen. John proposed and you accepted. You was over the moon, but then fell back into a sort of coma again. As for the ruckus outside, Mr Meigh dispersed the crowd. He got me and Joseph, the coachman, to put whatever coats and hats and scarfs that we could find and lay them over the backs of the chairs in the dining room. We didn't know what his plan was at first and thought 'ed gone bonkers like, but 'e edged the crowd over so they would be outside those winders and then 'e got the response 'e was looking for. One of them shouted out, 'Hay lads, owd up, 'ay's got a bliddy army in theer. Ay's trying to trick us', then they all started moving away, slowly at first, then the rain started up again and they scarpered off. We found you collapsed in the outhouse, brought you in here and Mr Meigh got the doctor for you."

"Thank you, Dinah."

"That's OK, I'll bring a spot of lunch for you later, if you're up to it, ducky." and Dinah left me alone with my thoughts.

God in heaven, what have I done? I must have been delirious, accepting John's proposal. I'd gone through such a trauma and John had been with me, protecting me all the while. Yes, he's a lovely guy, but do I love him enough to marry him, I mean, it was all so quick. Before getting out alive from the fiasco in Burslem, I hadn't even thought of him in that way. What if I do marry him, what will our future be? If I'm stuck in the 19th century and can never go back again, what will life be like, where will we live? I vaguely remembered Job Meigh saying something about getting us a cottage – but life in the 19th century was dire. I had only managed to stand it as Job Meigh had got all the new mod cons of the day in at Ash Hall – running water, gas and even the early flushing toilets, although no electricity as yet. The villagers around had none of that and even worse in Hanley and surrounding towns, with their stinking, sewerage-filled gutters and alleyways. But, who could blame them, there were no sewers.

It was gradually dawning on me that I'd made my bed and I had to lie in it – make the best of a bad job. There was no going back. Yes, I'd marry John. He was a nice guy, though very rough round the edges. Maybe I could smooth down those edges, calm down his Potteries dialect. In any case, he was good with his hands, maybe he could fit in running water and gas, and a flushing toilet into whatever cottage Job Meigh was going to rent to us.

I began to think of the comparative luxury I'd had in the 21st century – central heating, showers, baths, washing machines, computers, buying things on line, banking, cookers, microwaves, televisions, blue tooth, ipads, radio, ipods, telephones, smartphones, cars, flights – holidays, supermarkets, libraries, dentists, doctors, hospitals...... my head was spinning with the number of inventions, just for daily living, not including work-related inventions – and pensions, universities, colleges, training courses..... none of these were now available to me and it wasn't as if I knew how any of these inventions worked or could make, or get John to make, to make my life easier. I'd not had any training as an electrician or plumber or manufacturer – we just took all of these things for granted – go on line or round the shops and buy things – you didn't have to make them yourself, and it would be impossible to do so without the technology, skills, machinery, raw materials – I mean, steel hadn't even been invented,.... had it? Nor had plastic come to that, nor pneumatic tyres or the combustion engine - although, given 10 years or so and that might be on the horizon. There wasn't even a sewing machine. Come to think of it, I thought to myself, there must be steel - there are all these cotton mills and steel cages used in the coal mines – steel rolling mills, shaping molten steel into all different shapes and wire for thousands of different uses. Sheffield was the steel capital, making all sorts of knives and blades and tools. I suppose the world was waiting for the Bessemer converter to enable mass production of high quality steel to be produced.

But that still leaves me as a lone, lost female, in a man's world, where women are thought nothing of, unless they've inherited money, to be used as men desire, no vote, no say. It's not as though I could approach a steel rolling mill and ask them to make me a washing machine, eh? I started to laugh to myself at the thought. Then I started to cry. I didn't even have enough money to get myself a pair of shoes, so how could I approach a steel rolling mill and ask for them to invent a washing machine?

I thought back, or was it forward, to the 1950s, as I was growing up. Mum had an old free-standing boiler she did the washing in. It was electric but she had to fill it herself with water, which emptied from a spout at the bottom. The electricity turned a sort of plastic spinning device attached to the bottom of the boiler. This device had blades that would turn the washing. It would turn one way, then turn the other way through the centre of the boiler. Of course, that was run by electricity and the spinner was plastic, both of which weren't invented yet. I suppose, before that, they had to heat water over the fire and pour it into barrels and physically stir with a long pole, something I believe I recall, in the back of my mind, was called a dolly - and a device a bit like massive tweezers, made of wood with a rounded steel bracket at one end bolted to the wood. This would be used for stirring and getting the hot clothes out of the barrel. I suppose I'd have to do the same. Mum still used a wash board for some stained items. This was a corrugated piece of thick glass framed by wood. I remember the group 'the Skiffles' would use these wash boards as a musical instrument and anything else they could find that they could get a tune out of, one of which being 'My old man's a dustman', and I found myself singing the song. "Oh go away", I shouted to myself – "I don't want you running through my head!"

So, I resumed - what was I fit to do, work-wise? Yes, I could help stroke victims with exercise regimes. I could teach, a bit, but even geography would have changed, with countries having changed names and become independent. The past 170 years of history hadn't happened yet.

Oh, It was all just too much.

Just then John came in, walked over and gave me a kiss. "Well, mar leedy, ow at?"

"Oh, a bit better, John. We have a lot to talk about. I know I agreed to marry you.... and I will, but when, ...and where will we live?"

"Ah've spoken wi' Mr Meigh, just a quick word loik, as 'es aht doing 'is magistrate wark. The police 'en army 've bin rinding up the payple involved int' riots. Thusands of 'em. Thah've all gotten te go to trial. The trials are moestly tacking pleece in Casstle, 'cept fer t'Charteests, ef thee catch 'em.. 'E'll bay gone a couple of wayks or mur. Onyweeys, 'e said yer con steey 'ere fer t'arm baying. Yer nahs 'ah've bin building neuw 'owses for 'im on't esteeat. Mebbie way con 'ev one o' thim in a bit, wunct way're merit. Thah's nay rush, gee us tahm to get to know each uther better. Eet's o bin a bit o' a rush, may proposing en you accepting, although I nahs ah loves yer en ah dunna want te wayt tay leng to git marrit. Whut sess yer te spring, yer dunna want a winter wedding, doss yer? Eet'd gee us tahm to build th'owse, mack it just as yer'd loik it, running watter en o thut. What de yer seey?"

"That would be fine, John. It would give me time to sort myself out. Find another job that I can possibly do. Mrs Meigh doesn't need all that help now."

"Ah donno abite thet, mar love. Ah dunna want yer warking when way're merrit. Ah con provide fer yer, donna yer fayre. Eet wunna bay raight. En whin the childer come along, yer'll naid te bay 'om te looek efter 'em."

"Children, Oh I hadn't even thought of that. Oh well, if and when that happens, I'll stop home but, in the meantime, I would like to be busy, bring in a little bit of income so we can have the things we want to make life comfortable."

"Az yer weshes, lovely. Ah nows yer do things different loik dine sithe en ah wunna want yer to bay unhappy, but ah nayds a woif, who will bay thar fer may en the childer…. when thay comes. Ah suppose, az lung az yer loves may, way con wark things ite."

"Yes, John. I love you and will be there for you." And I reached up to give him a kiss. "Now I'm tired and wish to rest, so can I see you later?"

"Oraight, mar lovely. Git yer slayp. Way'll wark things ite." And John left the room, blowing me a kiss.

This all worried me even more. Children – excruciatingly painful childbirth with no drugs! God in heaven – and no contraceptives. Oh well,…. I suppose women have been doing it since Eve. What must be must be… but then again, a lot of women died in childbirth…..At that, I dozed off for a fitful sleep.

CHAPTER 2 – THE AFTERMATH

There was a flicker in John's eyes and he was moving his lips but no sound was coming out. "Don't try to talk, John. You've had a heart attack at the pit. I got you brought back here. You'll be a bit uncomfortable as you're lying on a door some lads brought you in on. When you're a bit better, I'll get it removed, but in the meantime, just lie there. I don't want you to move. I've got you some tea and some soup, if you can take it.

I managed to cradle John's head in my lap and lift him up a bit so he could sup on the warm camomile tea, followed by a few spoonfuls of soup. He gave a few groans while feeding him, but his eyes were closed. He was automatically feeding, like a baby. When he didn't respond to anymore spoonfuls, I rested his head gently back down again and let him sleep.

There'd still been no report back from the pit. I didn't know whether or not Alfred had been found and brought out. I was sure someone would tell me if they'd found him. He was stll my baby, even though he was grown up with a family of his own, and I felt so helpless. I'd tried desperately to change his mind and get another job. He was intelligent, capable, there were other jobs out there, but he wanted to be with his pals, to feel one of the lads. There were so many pit explosions and so many young lads, men – and women – who had lost their lives in this dangerous career, it was a regular event. But I could do nothing about it but resign myself to the fact that, one day, sooner or later, I'd get the news that Alfred was badly injured, or even killed. I just waited and prayed each day that that day would not be the one. I'd done all my crying, or so I'd thought, as the tears started yet again. But John was my main worry now and I'd try my best to help him recover, to come back to me. I had to be strong for him.

I tried to get the thought out of my mind of Alfred, lying injured, up to his neck in water, with the searing blackness of the pit smothering him - crying out for help, trying to move, but not able to, as his broken bones denied him that. I offered up an ardent prayer for his safety. I'd never been that religious before but there are times when nothing else seems fitting, when there's nothing else left, nothing to grab hold of. "Oh God, please help Alfred and all the other people lying injured, dying. Please help those trying to find them. Please help John. Please accept those that have died into your kingdom and protect them." That's the only thing John and I had differed on when we had been together – religion. He was Methodist and I was basically no longer a believer. I did bring the children up to go to church though, as I felt they should know about the teachings and stories, from which they could learn the morals of life. I felt I had to attend as well, as I would be seen to be someone not to be trusted, if I didn't attend - Methodism was rife in the county. I would just sit in church, with the children, and John, as a family, and I'd think of other things. I believed also, that this was something missing from the future as certain people, who had missed these stories, I felt, lacked the moral judgement needed to get them through life. Of course, it was the same in any day and age – corrupt people doing whatever con tricks they could to get money – to steal from the innocent, the poor and the elderly, those unable to defend themselves, for their own gain. There would always be that element in society, no matter what faith they had been brought up in.

My thoughts strayed back to Alfred, but no, I had to get my mind off the pit disaster, and that horrendous hallucination of drowning in the black-inky ocean, and back to John, someone I could help, otherwise all would be lost, I'd be lost to myself, caught up in my own distress, in utter turmoil and I'd be no help to anyone. I had to be strong for John.

I began to think about the time after the riots, when I was taken dreadfully ill myself. "That was a bad time but it's when I accepted your proposal, John" I found myself saying out loud. "Of course a lot has changed since then and a lot of water has passed under the bridge, as you know."

I saw John's eyes open, and he looked at me. He tried to move and say something. "Oh John, you'll be alright soon. Don't worry, I'm here with you. Just take it easy and rest awhile" I could see him relax a bit - so, he could hear me and seemed to know what I was saying. That was a relief in itself. "We've had our ups and downs over the years but you could never get your head around my secret. I should have told you right from the start but I daren't." I saw John's eyes twitch and he was beginning to look stressed. He'd opened his eyes and was trying to move his hand but just the fingers moved. "Oh, I know John, I shouldn't be saying this sort of thing when you're so ill. I don't mean to stress you even more, but it's something that needs to be said. ...." I waited a while until John had calmed a bit, then against my better judgement, I continued. "I thought you'd think me cracked in the head, which, you did indeed think when you eventually found out. I'm so sorry you found out in the way you did and forgive me for talking about it now, when you're a sort of captive listener, but it's just that I've not been able to prove otherwise and you wouldn't listen." John gave a sort of a moan. I checked his pulse – it was racing a bit. "Oh John, you still think you married a witch or I'd come under the devil's influence. Anyway, you left me, John.... and I don't blame you. I should never have married you. I'm just really grateful for the time we had together and that you didn't blurt out my story to anyone who would listen. So, you saved my dignity, which meant I could carry on working and be respected by the community. It was a lot to ask but I dread to think what would have happened to me should the story have been broadcast. They'd probably have hung me or put me in a mental asylum. I'm not mental John. I've tried to tell you what the future is going to be like, all the inventions, the changes of government, the laws passed. I don't see how I could have made this all up, but you still think I have. It's not as though it's your immediate future, so I could tell you what was around the corner for you, and you'd believe me when it came to pass – but you wouldn't believe me, even then. So, we had to part." I let him rest after blurting this all out.

Imagine if Job Meigh, at Ash Hall, had got hold of the story, what with him being a magistrate. He would have had me stripped, whipped and drowned like the witches of old. I suppose you knew that, so you kept quiet. "You must have had a little bit of love in your heart for me, maybe you still do." I saw John's eyes closing again. "There John, go back to sleep. I'll be here when you wake up."

While John slept, my thoughts continued with Job Meigh. He was the pottery entrepreneur who built Ash Hall in 1837 and bought up most of the surrounding farms. Ash Hall is a mansion, on an elevated site, overlooking the Bucknall and Hanley, areas of Stoke. Job Meigh had managed to construct something that is incomparable to anything else in the area, perfectly adapted to every purpose of domestic comfort at the time. Adorning the front is an elegant portico, which comprises three beautiful Gothic arches, turreted and embattled, procuring gasps of amazement to anyone gazing upon it. The exterior is of hard stone, retrieved from the estate, of an ash colour, giving the building a mistaken feeling of antiquity, with oriel windows, surmounted with pediments or pointed gables which harmonise with the style of the architecture, being that of a Gothic manor house construction,. The adjoining lawn is tastefully laid out and planted; and, altogether, one of the most beautiful buildings I've seen.

Job had worked out of the Old Hall Pottery in Hanley, Staffordshire from 1805, producing high quality stone and earthenware. He had married Elizabeth, daughter of William Mellor of Johnson's Charles Street Pottery in Hanley, in 1805. He and his brother-in-law, Richard Hicks, who had married Job's sister, Lydia in 1801, bought a factory in Broad Street, Hanley and rebuilt the works. It was said to have consisted of 60 rooms, seven ovens and five offices. At one time they had 600 people working there and I'd heard that the works were well run and the hours were fewer than in some other works – that is, in summer from six to six and, in winter, from seven to six. In other works some of the children, called cutters, attending the printers, appeared to me to be extremely tired. They were required to attend in the morning one hour before the printer, to light fires and prepare the area for the day's work, and often had to wait in the evening, for some time after the rest had departed, to prepare for the next day. The cutter-girls and plate-maker boys, from 8 years old, or even less, made up a 5th of the workforce.

At the time, Job Meigh lived in an elegant mansion house at the top of Albion Street, before moving to Ash Hall, He was known for his philanthropy and liberality, justly regarded as one of the worthies of the district, to whom people referred to for his confidence and strict impartial decisions. Job Meigh had been one of the first to set up the New Connexion Methodism, with other New Connexion Methodist, namely William Smith, and George and John Ridgway, putting money up, to extend the Bethesda Church in Hanley – religious scenes were also common in Meigh's work. In 1859 a colonnade was added to the front of the chapel, with a window and cornice above, designed by Staffordshire architect Robert Scrivener. Job's most well-known and popular works were white stoneware jobs with relief decoration of Gothic Revival motifs – so that's where I presume his inspiration for the Gothic style of Ash Hall came from. In 1823 His Royal Highness, the Duke of Sussex, presented the gold Medal of the Society of Arts to him, for having given to the public a Glaze for Common Pottery, entirely free from the deleterious qualities of the usual lead glaze.

Charles, his younger brother, continued this business, going into business with his son, also called Charles, in 1850. He exhibited at the Great Exhibition of 1851 and in 1886 won a medal.

Yes, he certainly had taste but not the sort of person you wanted to cross, as I discovered when I found myself working for him back in 1842, looking after his wife, who had suffered a stroke following a brain haemorrhage. He may have been philanthropic and liberal to the outside world, having saved my John, following a severe bout of depression. John's, first wife had died, and John had become so depressed, he was incapable of working, and subsequently homeless and on the street. Job Meigh had found him and had given him a job, on the estate, to work at his own rate until he was better. Yes, Job Meigh had a kind side, when he wanted, but he definitely showed signs of misogyny – women weren't to be trusted and were only good for one thing. That was, basically, the common view of women in Stoke, at the time, and possibly in the whole of the world. He definitely had a temper on in him and could snap like the click of your fingers into a different, violent person. After looking after his wife for a time, John had told me the real story behind Elizabeth Meigh's stroke. It seems that Job Meigh and his wife had a violent quarrel as their horse and carriage pulled up at the hall. John had seen Job push Elizabeth out of the carriage, head-first, onto frozen January ground. Elizabeth never fully recovered but, following my programme of exercises and assistance with her speech, she made great strides and was able to mingle with company again. Before my coming, she had basically locked herself in her room. She never forgave her husband.

Of course, John Meigh had sold the factory before I came on the scene but I remember getting to speak to one of the boys at Job Meigh's old factory, one time – Charles Hall. Mr Ridgway, another New Connexion Methodist, had come to visit Job Meigh. Mr Ridgway had taken over the factory with his partners Mr Morley and Mr Wear. Mr Ridgway had left some vital paperwork at the hall when he visited, so I took the opportunity to take this to him. Charles Hall was just 9 years old. He had been employed at the factory for six months and worked from 6am to 6pm in the summer and from 7am to 6pm in the winter. He had a break of half an hour for breakfast, which consisted of tea with bread and butter, plus a one hour break for dinner of beef and potatoes. He admitted that he was very tired at the end of the day but, when I asked him if he liked to go to work at the factory, he answered "yes". His pay was two shillings and three pence a week and he confirmed that there were separate water closets for the boys and girls. He had formerly been to school and could read and write and now went to a Sunday school.

I also managed to speak to another employee, Alice Berrisford, who was aged 17 at the time. She'd been working at the factory for six years. She too had been to school, could read and write and now went to a Sunday school. She worked the same hours as Charles hall but added that, on Saturday, work stopped at 4pm. Her pay was 4 shillings a week and she had a sister, who was also employed at the factory.

....

Thinking about what Job Meigh would have done to me, if he ever found out my secret, reminded me of the court cases following the Pottery riots on 15th and 16th August 1842. I had been to a few after I'd recovered enough to attend.

John and I had been following the rioters and had hid behind the garden wall at the Big House in Burslem as thousands more of starving people entered the town from Moorlands Avenue, coming from Macclesfield and Leek. They met the army, on horseback, and the special police, in a stand-off, outside the Big House. Lt.

Col Thomas Powys had read the riot act, telling the crowd to go home peacefully, but the crowd were not moving, shouting out that they had nothing to go home to, except starvation. When the crowd started throwing stones, Joseph Heapy had been the first to be shot. He'd been standing right by the wall of the Big House, possibly just an on-looker, but one person in the army saw him bend down, looking like he was about to pick up a stone to throw, and turned his rifle on him, shooting him through the head.

I had made a special effort to attend the inquest of Josiah Heapy, the poor man who was shot in front of the Big House in Burslem, while John and I were hiding, behind the garden wall, scared for our lives, frightened to even breathe in case we were discovered and shot too. The inquest was held by the Burslem Coroner, William Harding. He described examining the body and finding a mortal wound on the upper part of the head. The skull was shattered and the brain protruding. He was of the opinion that it was the result of a gunshot, and that death was instantaneous. Heapy was found with 3s 5d in his pockets, in silver and copper. A young woman came forward and identified herself as Sarah Heapy, a cousin of the deceased. She told the inquest that he was an apprentice shoemaker, aged nineteen, from Leek, employed by Mr Rigby of Market Place, Leek. She said he was a widower, whose wife had died just two weeks earlier, and he had three children. She claimed he was forced on the march to the Potteries, along with her three brothers. In further evidence, she claimed he had put twenty sovereigns in his trouser watch pocket, which he had collected for a Rechabite Society he belonged to. The coroner then asked for the body to be checked again, in view of the jury. No money or watch pocket were found. Sarah Heapy was now questioned in more detail about the money and claimed to have seen the deceased place the money on a table on Tuesday morning, whereupon she counted them. As no money could be found, the coroner cast doubt on her whole story and he was not satisfied with the evidence. A juror stood up and commented that Heapy, had he been forced to join the mob, did not have to throw stones or lead from the front as some witnesses had claimed he had. The coroner now asked the jury to bring in a verdict, and quite quickly returned with "justifiable homicide".

I still had the newspapers I had bought at the time. They'd gone a bit faded now, but I had kept them safe in box. I started rummaging through them.

I found an interesting letter that appeared in the Staffordshire Advertiser a couple of days later. Josiah Heapy's brother wrote stating that the person who called herself Sarah Heapy, and represented herself as a cousin of the deceased was incorrect from beginning to end. The brother stated that Heapy was never married, that he was a quiet, sober, and an inoffensive youth. He was totally unconnected with any political party, and was forced away from Leek, by the crowd, against his will. The writer also stated that Heapy's master, Mr Rigby, also speaks of him in the highest terms. So, clearly, Sarah Heapy was an impostor and had been looking for a reward of some kind for her evidence. I remember thinking at the time that Heapy had been young to be married and have three children by the age of 19, but then again, that was the era when people had large families. So, had there been 20 sovereigns and would she have been given them if they had been found?

In the Bolton Chronicle a report suggested that the cause of the riots was "the apathy of the church authorities. The Dissenters, but most especially a sect called the Kilhamites, or Wesleyan New Connexion, of which Mr Ridgway, of Anti Corn Law League notoriety, is a member. It went on to claim that the religious education of these towns had been left entirely to these new religions and, as a result, the working classes had been thoroughly steeped in radicalism." The same correspondent also felt that the Potteries was unjustified in rioting as it was suffering less than any other place in the Midlands or North. I remember remarking at the time that Job Meigh was a New Connexion follower and wondered what he thought about that statement.

Anyway, all public meetings of Chartists were banned by the magistrates. The large build-up of troops in the area meant it was now quiet, and people were not even troubled by intimidating beggars. The large number of troops in the area had the effect of giving the impression that Stoke and surrounding areas were under the state of martial Law. The remaining military in the area were a troop of 2nd Dragoons, three companies of 34th infantry, two companies of 12 infantry, and five troops of Staffordshire Yeomanry Cavalry.

By now the roundups of known Chartists and rioters had begun. All week following the riots two courts a day were sitting in Newcastle - one in the Town Hall and the other at the Police Station. The courts were manned by a team of magistrates working in rota, amongst whom were Thomas Hartshorne, John Harvey, Job Meigh and Captain Mainwaring. Each day prisoners had been brought into Newcastle from the surrounding district until, by the end of the first week, several hundred had been seen by the magistrates and either released or punished and, for the more serious cases, committed for trial at Stafford Assizes. The Staffordshire Advertiser commented that many of those taken in front of the magistrates seemed to show no sorrow for their action, "which clearly showed how deeply their minds were perverted by the infatuating influence which had taken possession of them". I read further.... By Friday, 19th August 1842 641 prisoners were in Stafford Goal awaiting trial.

I remember seeing one of the trials taken by Job Meigh and Captain Mainwaring, in Newcastle. I'd made notes at the time and retrieved these from the box. It was Samuel Robinson on the stand. He was charged with using seditious language and incitement to riot. Someone called Mathew Horrobin had been giving evidence about others charged and he was called again as the main witness against Robinson. On oath he stated that he saw Robinson, on the Monday, 15th August 1842, directing people to different houses, and instructing which to destroy and what to burn. When Robinson was asked what he had to say, he told the court that in fact all the troubles had been caused by Anti Corn Law League agitators. Robinson claimed he had tried to stop the destruction but he had been unable to speak to the mob. He then said that he went away, claiming that the Chartists cause would be injured for five years by the rioting. Mr R Daniel, of Stoke, then offered to stand bail for Robinson to the amount of £2000. (I remember thinking this was a huge sum at the time). This was refused by the magistrates, who considered the evidence against him too serious. So, this case would have gone onto Stafford for trial. I couldn't help thinking that Samuel Robinson was probably culpable as I hadn't seen anyone at the time, actually trying to stop the rioters, though maybe John and I, as we followed the rioters, weren't where he was.

Others charged included a man called Neal, known amongst the local Chartists as "Home Secretary". A person named Kimber was nearly sent to goal on the ground thet he had been talking to soldiers on duty and at their barracks. The only thing which saved him from gaol was that the magistrates gave him the benefit of the doubt as they were unsure of his motives.

Elizabeth Poulson and Samuel Wilshaw were charged with stealing pledges from Mr Hall, pawnbroker, at Hanley on Tuesday, 16th. As they had later returned them, they were both discharged. This had in fact become quite common as a method of trying to avoid prosecution.

Thomas Owen, a labourer from Shelton, was charged with rioting at Rev Aikins' property on 15th. He was seen coming out of the house when it was on fire, with his face blackened and was heard to say, "We are the boys that can do it." Neither John nor I had been at Rev Aikins to see the destruction. We were ensconced in the relative safety of the George and Dragon when we heard news that a lot of drunken rioters were revelling in the destruction they'd carried out. More beer and wines had been found and the desperate men who drank them were ready for any villainy. The house was set on fire and its contents destroyed. Thomas Owen was identified as the leader of the mob at Mr Parker's house too, and was committed for trial.

Edward Smith, a clog and pattern-maker, was seen in one of the bedrooms of the house, knocking the window sashes out, and then throwing furniture out onto the fire in front of the house. He too was committed for trial. He, along with Samuel Tildsley, who was charged with breaking the windows in Burslem Town Hall on the night of 16th August, was sent for trial. Richard Croxton, accused of taking seven sovereigns from Mr Meigh's foreman, by intimidation, had a witness swear against him, saying that Croxton had stated, "I ought to have had three times seven sovereigns, for I could have caused the bloody place to have been burnt down." He also made a remark about, "walking up to his knees in blood", which can hardly have impressed the magistrates. One prisoner, Dennis Mulligan, was quoted as saying to the court, in a broad Irish accent, "It was not a glass I was drinking out of, gentlemen, it was a bacon dish!" and laughing out loud.

Matthew Horrobin was called again to give evidence against Thomas Lester. Horrobin's evidence this time, was that Lester had attended a small meeting of about thirty men in a field at the back of Keeling's Lane in Hanley. A list was brought to the meeting by a man called Gilbert, and read out. It contained the names of several prominent local people and Gilbert called for their houses to be burnt down. This was put to the meeting as a motion and no-one objected. This was enough evidence to send Lester for trial. I couldn't help querying to myself, by this time, why this guy was being called up so many times to give evidence – surely he couldn't have been in loads of different places at the same time? Was there something more to this – did he or someone else hold a grudge against these people and were willing to pay Horrobin to perjure himself? Much of the evidence was at best hearsay, and often inconclusive.

I attended the court the next day as the session concerned the demolishing of Dr Vale's premises on 15th August. I had been there with John. Dr Vale was the rector of Longton. The mob arrived about 2pm. Dr Vale's wife had attempted to calm the crowd at first but they soon discovered the rector's cellars. Crowds of females, with the greatest eagerness, pushed forward to partake, among others, of the liquor. We saw a man bringing out the alcohol, which the women, and others in the crowd, surged forward to grab hold of. One woman had poured alcohol into a pint basin, saying to her companions, "'ere wenches, drink. Thah's plentah mer". The mob had got themselves so drunk they could not stand to run away and were staggering all over the place. One woman was fortunate to escape by being placed in a wheelbarrow by friends and removed. The rector's furniture and his valuable collection of rare books were hoisted onto a bonfire, lit in front of the house. Furniture, in turn, was thrown out of the windows onto the fire. We saw someone demolishing the woodwork surrounding the windows while others were breaking up bedroom furniture by banging the pieces together. Then the house itself was set alight. I heard someone remark, "Ay well deserved that. Eet woz 'im who mayed the crass remark abite 'ow way poor payple should use grass en leaves te mack tay ef way codna afford to bay it fer th' shops. Good reedance t'im, thut's whut ah says." Anyway, a fire engine arrived, followed by the 2nd dragoons and managed to save the structure of the house. Some of the previous by-standers actually started assisting the fire brigade. Prisoners were taken.

I found out more at the court session. A group of ten men and women were escorted into the courtroom, each charged with rioting and demolishing the property at Dr Vale's on 15th August. Richard Wright was the one who set fire to the house, with a firebrand, which he applied to a heap of broken furniture in one of the rooms. This man, along with Thomas Jackson, William Hollins and Mary Shaw, were seen throwing furniture on a fire in front of the house. James Earp was seen demolishing the woodwork around the windows, whilst Joseph and Philip Saunders were seen breaking bedroom furniture by banging the pieces together. The prisoner, Rosanna Ellis, along with Millicent Saunders, was seen carrying alcohol, which a man had brought from the cellar, in a pint basin, saying to her companions, "'Ere wenches, drink. Thah's plentah mer". Another prisoner, Elizabeth Robinson was seen carrying a bundle of clothes, covered with a while dimity petticoat. They were all sent for trial.

Jeremiah Yates, potter and keeper of a coffee shop near Miles Bank, was next. He was charged with being one of a party who turned out the workmen at the factory of Messrs. Ridgway, Morley & Co., in Shelton, on Monday, 15th. We'd seen a large meeting of colliers at Ridgway's coal mine, while making our way back to the George and Dragon. The meeting had seemed to be quiet and orderly so we stopped a while to listen. Mr Ridgway was holding a meeting of his own to discuss the workers' grievances and offer moderation. I remember John telling me that Ridgway was one of the few reasonable pit owners, paying fair wages and looking after the welfare of the sick under his charge. However, at that moment, we heard the sound of people and horses approaching. Sneyd, a local magistrate and coal owner, approached at the head of cavalry and infantry, ordering the crowd to disperse. Mr Ridgway requested the right to continue the meeting but Sneyd ignored this request and read the Riot Act. This led to an uproar by the crowd of miners, obviously taken aback as they hadn't been doing any harm and had not been out of order, just quietly listening to their boss' counsel. However, Sneyd wasn't having this. He stated that he had orders not to allow any crowd meetings, no matter how calm and controlled, and sent the infantry forward to arrest all in the crowd.. That's when John and I made a quick getaway. Two witnesses were presented at court, Thomas Furnival and John Lawton, who both gave evidence against Yates and he was sent for trial, although he was fortunate in being released on bail first. This didn't make any sense to me. There was no turn-out at Ridgways'. The miners were calm and collected in discussion with Ridgway until Sneyd came along. Who were these two witnesses? Were they another two, who had been paid to give false witness against Jeremiah Yates? Did someone have a grudge against him and wanted him out of the way? Something was definitely wrong in the kingdom of Denmark. It was beginning to look like the middle and upper classes had decreed that "something must be done". They were obviously clearly shocked and scared by the revolution, which had so nearly overpowered them, that anybody, who had the slightest suggestion of involvement in the troubles was to be severely punished.

They were definitely out for the Chartist speakers. I heard later that Capper was easily picked up. He had been there with the other Chartists on 15th August 1842. He had been urging all the thousands gathered there to seek their rights, but by peaceable means. He had continued that it was the opinion of the meeting that nothing but the People's Charter could give the populace the power to have a fair day's wage for a fair day's work. However, he was said to have stated, according to the papers "Those who cannot afford to get guns must get pikes, and those who cannot afford to get either must get torches." Obviously he denied saying this, and neither John nor I, when attending the Chartist gatherings, heard anything by any of the Chartist speakers about taking up arms. It was their aim to strike, yes, but peacefully, and they tried to press this home to the crowds attending that any show of aggression would weaken their cause to get the People's Charter accepted. So, again, there were witnesses giving false statements. Claims by the Chartist speakers that these witnesses were false, fell on deaf ears. Joseph Capper was arrested by four men on Sunday evening, August 21st 1842, on a charge of seditious speaking. As opposed to Frith, a local draper and tailor, who was to be a main witness against Joseph Capper at his subsequent trial and the supposed aggressive statements made by Capper, it seems that Capper, who was an old man, (according to Charles Shaw, reporter at the time), "quietly surrendered to his captors. He presented a perfect contrast to the tumult and excitement which prevailed as he was led through the marketplace, past his own workshop, his old wife and son and daughter following, accompanied by a sympathetic crowd". Capper was taken to Newcastle-under-Lyme for 'safety'. 'Who's safety was this', I asked myself, 'Capper's or the town of Tunstall's?' I suppose the authorities were worried that the gangs of men still wandering the district at this time would quickly have formed a plan to secure the freedom of this popular leader from any lock up in Tunstall or Burslem. After all, they had freed three miners held accused of vagrancy in Burslem just a couple of weeks earlier.

John Richards was soon picked up and brought to Newcastle for his committal. John and I had seen him at the Crown Bank in Hanley on the morning of 15th August 1842, proposing that all labour must cease until the People's Charter becomes the law. Richards was known locals as 'Daddy Richards' and was seventy at the time of his arrest. The Staffordshire Advertiser reported the evidence against Richards with the opening words, "a long-winded speaker at most of the Chartist meetings". Still, he could pull a good crowd and the court was quite packed. James Goostry, the police officer, who had arrested Richards on a charge of seditious speaking, told the court that, when Richards had been shown the warrant for his arrest, he had stated that, whilst the warrant was a legal one, the charge was false. Richards, in his defence, stated that he had in fact been at Mr Fenton's, the pawnbroker, where he had helped to defend the property, with success. He was committed to Stafford for trial.

There were all sorts of reports at the time about Richards, even bringing Lord Palmerston into the picture. Richards, it seems, had become a follower of David Urquhart, who later became MP for Stafford – a radical sect that wanted to expose what they saw as a conspiracy between Lord Palmerston and Russian foreign agents. Urquhart believed that a plot had been hatched in 1839 in which twenty towns were to be seized by one hundred thousand armed Chartists. The Chartists were organised in cells of ten men, with a Council of Five at the top, with leaders which included a top police official. Urquhart was rather paranoid, and believed that such an efficient organisation could only be Russian. He compounded this with the belief that a Russian fleet was ready to set sail to Britain as soon as the revolution began. Urquhart, when he was informed of the planned uprising, quickly convinced two members of the Council of Five of the stupidity of their plan and, aided by twenty followers, put a stop to it. Unfortunately, as he told it, the messenger sent to Newport arrived too late to prevent the trouble there. Urquhart went on to convince a number of Chartist leaders that "every diplomat's closet contained a Russian", and Lord Palmerston was "a paid tool of St. Petersburg and every European cabinet was a nest of Russian-dominated mercenaries". So, not surprising that Richards lost support locally.

Still, I thought to myself while re-reading these reports, nothing has changed over the years. Apart from the Cold War, there had been uproar about the Russians on 4 March 2018, having poisoned a father and daughter, Sergei and Yulia Skripal, in Salisbury. Sergei was a former Russian military officer and double agent for the UK's intelligence services. They were poisoned with a Novichok nerve agent. After three weeks in a critical condition. Yulia regained consciousness and was able to speak. Her father regained consciousness one month later. A police officer was also taken into intensive care after being contaminated when he went to Sergei Skripal's house. Sergei had settled in the UK in 2010 following a spy swap. He held dual Russian and British Citizenship. His daughter was a Russian citizen and was visiting her father from Moscow. The British government accused Russia of attempted murder and announced a series of punitive measures against Russia, including the expulsion of diplomats. This was supported by 28 other countries. Russia, naturally, denied these accusations and expelled foreign diplomats - accusing Britain of the poisoning. On 30 June 2018 a similar poisoning of two British nationals in Amesbury, seven miles from Salisbury, involved the same nerve agent. A man found the nerve agent in a perfume bottle and gave it to a woman who sprayed it on her wrist. The woman, fell ill within 15 minutes and died on 8 July, but, fortunately, the man who also came into contact with the poison survived. British police believe this incident was not a targeted attack, but a result of the way the nerve agent was disposed of after the poisoning in Salisbury. On 5 September 2018, British authorities identified two Russian nationals, using the names Alexander Petrov and Ruslan Boshirov, as suspected of the Skripals' poisoning, and alleged that they were active officers in Russian military intelligence. In response, on 13 September, the two men were interviewed on Russian television, where they claimed they were businessmen and tourists visiting the city. The media commented afterwards upon inconsistencies in their descriptions. For example, they claimed to have planned a holiday long in advance, whereas their flights were actually booked "at the last minute", and the brevity of their stay counter-stated their claims.

British Prime Minister, Theresa May, announced in the Commons that British intelligence services had identified the two suspects as officers in the GU Intelligence Service (formerly known as GRU) and the assassination attempt was not a rogue operation and was "almost certainly" approved at a senior level of the Russian government. May also said Britain would push for the EU to agree new sanctions against Russia.

Prime Minister, Theresa May, said in the House of Commons that it was now clear that Mr Skripal and his daughter were poisoned with a military-grade nerve agent of a type developed by Russia. Russia's record of conducting state-sponsored assassinations; and our assessment that Russia views some defectors as legitimate targets for assassinations; the Government has concluded that it is highly likely that Russia was responsible for the act against Sergei and Yulia Skripal. She added that there were therefore only two plausible explanations for what happened in Salisbury on the 4th of March. Either this was a direct act by the Russian State against our country, or the Russian government had lost control of this potentially catastrophically damaging nerve agent and allowed it to get into the hands of others. May also requested that Russia explain which of these two possibilities it was. If there was no credible response, the government would conclude that this amounted to unlawful use of force by the Russian State against the United Kingdom and an ultimatum would be put to Putin. Russia did not come back with an account so the 23 Russian intelligence agents were expelled and countermeasures put into action.

The White House also accused Russia of undermining the security of countries worldwide.

The Russian foreign ministry spokesperson, speaking on a Russian state television channel on the evening of 13 March, said that no one had the right to present Russia with 24-hour ultimatums.

Finally, the poisoning has been officially declared to be a fabrication and a "grotesque provocation rudely staged by the British and U.S. intelligence agencies" to undermine Russia.

"Oh, those bloody Russians", went through my head – words from a song by Boney M.

Anyway, that was enough of what the future held, and I returned to my notes on the trials of the Chartists.

Richards, it seems, was distinctly upset by hearing the fate of his comrade Chartists. In the Northern Star the following week, he complained that families have been left destitute, and that he has not one farthing with which to relieve them, or help his friends Oldham, Robinson and Yates. He went on, "My head is ready to split with pain, my heart almost at bursting, and when I reflect on the cause, and see the goodly fabric of Chartism thrown down in these parts, my soul sinks within me and I feel completely unmanned" and finished, "... should this vile aristocratic move succeed and the chains of slavery be riveted on the neck of my country, then farewell hope, farewell friends, farewell life, for to live in slavery and no hope will kill me outright." I thought to myself that there must be a poet in the man to express himself so whistfully, to say the least, but definitely heartfelt. I'd seen the despair and oppression which ordinary men lived under, first hand, and it is easy enough to see why they were driven to the lengths of this revolution, even though it was unplanned.

On delving further into the box, I found newspaper reports. Luckily Dinah had saved all the old papers for me, as she knew how interested I was in the news, and I'd stored them in my box so many years ago. One report was from Queen Victoria herself. She is quoted on 17th August as having written to Sir Robert Peel, the Prime Minister, and Sir James Graham, the Home Secretary, stating how surprised she was by the way the authorities had presented so little opposition to the rioters in the Potteries and "the passiveness of the troops". She felt that, apprehending Cooper and the other Manchester delegates must be a priority. Sir Robert Peel replied that, "every vigilance will be exerted with reference to Thomas Cooper and all the other itinerant agitators".

Thomas Cooper had been the main speaker when we were at the Crown Bank on 14th and 15th August 1842, leading the crowd in Chartist hymns. I remembered one of them:

Men of England, ye are slaves
Bought by tyrants, sold by knaves;
Your's the toil, the sweat, the pain,
Their's the profit, ease, and gain.

Men of England, ye are slaves;
Beaten by policemen's staves;
If their force ye dare repel
Your's will be the felon's cell.

Men of England, ye are slaves;
Hark! The stormy tempest raves
'Tis the nation's voice I hear
Shouting, "Liberty is near!"

Cooper was well able to address the thousands at the meeting, with his booming voice transcending the crowd. He was a man in his mid 30s – dark, wavy hair swept back from his high forehead, reaching to just about his shoulders. His lips were full and red and he would have been handsome if it were not for a small chin. He had eyes that gave the appearance of an energetic man, but also passionate and caring; however, these same eyes had the ability to penetrate and crowd and mesmerise. The crowd hung on his every word.

So, Queen Victoria had got the ball rolling and Thomas Cooper, was arrested within a couple of days, in Leicester, and brought back to the Potteries, then taken to Newcastle for a hearing. I had gone along. Cooper was charged with "exciting a multitude to riot and make a great noise. It wasn't Job Meigh this time as the examining magistrate, but Captain Mainwaring and J A Wise Esq. They were told by witnesses that Cooper's words, " Peace, law and order" had been said not in earnest, but in innuendo. Cooper argued whether he could really be convicted of the crime of innuendo, conveniently ignoring the effect he must have known his words could have on the crowd. (A good point, I thought while sitting there in the courtroom – he sounded like he had a legal background). The magistrates also wondered whether they could examine a bundle of papers brought with Cooper from Leicester, as these had not been specified on the warrant. He was committed to Stafford for trial on a charge of aiding a riot at Hanley. He was kept at Newcastle overnight, awaiting transportation the next day to Stafford.

That's what I thought was the end of that - he would be simply taken to Stafford and sentenced there - but word got around the next day that Cooper was to be borne away in an open carriage drawn by four horses, accompanied by a troop of cavalry, having drawn sword, taking him to Whitmore station. At Whitmore, the constable accompanying him, handcuffed his wrist and took him on the train to Stafford. Had this been to prevent an attack? It seems the carriage had passed by an area known locally as 'Higherland' (Ireland), due to the number of Irish labourers, who generally supported Feargus O'Connor, the Irish leader of Chartism. The officials were worried that the Irish would either try to free him or harm him as a suspected informer.

Anyway, Cooper got safely to Stafford gaol, along with a total of over seven hundred other prisoners, a mixture of Chartists and common criminals.

We'd seen William Ellis on 16th August 1842, encouraging the crowd to continue until the Charter became the law of the land. He was the main person out of the Chartists, who had roused the crowd. We'd heard him shouting to the crowd at the top of his voice, "Now me lads, we have got the parson's house down, we must have the churches down, for if we lose this day, we lose the day forever..... so now lads, for Burslem and now to business." That's when the crowd started on the move in a massive procession, led by women, in the direction of Burslem. So, in my mind, if any of the Chartists should have been at fault for the riots, it was him.

Delving in my box again, it appeared that, on 17th August, a letter was sent from a Burslem JP to the Home Secretary suggesting "it would be a most important step to get Ellis out of the way as he does a vast deal of harm. He was one of the mob which attacked the military and obliged them to fire." The letter went on to show the evidence given, under oath, by John Williams, a grocer from Sandbach. In that deposition he claimed that Ellis told his audience, at a meeting on Crown Bank, on 16th August, that, "There is only one soldier for every hundred inhabitants in the United Kingdom, and that, if the Chartists did not obtain political freedom before the Red Coats returned from China and India, they would be thrown back a hundred years." In a note by the Home Secretary, it was stated that "Ellis should be caught immediately. If, after the words spoken by him, he took an active part in resisting the military, the case assumes the character of treason, at all event he is guilty of a high misdemeanour."

CHAPTER 3 – THE REFORM BILL

After the Pottery riots an aura of depression prevailed for some years. The People's Charter had been refused, yet again, by the Government. There was a sullen, passive reign of distrust among the people. The Reform Bill had disappointed them. All their trade conflicts had ended in failure. Even the resounding attacks against the Corn Laws, then beginning to fill the country, excited little interest among the working classes, and so they gave little response. Betrayal and failure had made them sad and hopeless. Other industrial areas seemed to be getting on better but the Potteries people seemed to lack assertion. They returned to their seemingly feudal ties, landlord and serf.

I remember I was out on my rounds as a nurse one day, visiting Jimmy, who had been in a fight.

"How did you get into this state?" I asked him.

"Aw, the bailiff, was cracking on abite not rimembering mar neeme as 'e 'ardly says may. Well, ah gives 'im a luk as such – donna want te touch 'im, or 'ed ah'geen may wot fer, but ah was mad loik. Ah maynes, ah comes in loik everyone else, when ah feels loik eet. Wayre all t'sem. Eet's the way eet is. Onyways, ah wus mad en fanged olt of a pleete somwon 'ad just feneshed, en brock eet. 'Cos the geezer jest lamped may one, en way got in a scuffle. Bailiff jest looks on – dinna stop us."

So I ascertained from this that there was little in the way of discipline in the pot-banks, which differentiated them from the industrial workers of Lancashire and Yorkshire, areas where machinery and mechanisation was beginning to stamp itself into everyday work. Machinery meant discipline – workers had to work to strict hours, with cost of production bearing heavily on the amount produced, with labour being heavily monitored by overseers. You couldn't just close down a machine because so and so hadn't turned up. However, there was no such introduction of heavy machinery in the Potteries, and no effective economical management of the pot-works.

Jimmy continued, "Ah was surpraised to say bailiff thar. Ah mayne, 'e 'ardly ever comes rined. Thought ah'd bay able te snake in. Ah mayne, ah'd 'ad a skinful the night afore en codna git outa mar pit. Jest thought ah'd come in, di mar bit en mack up fer eet next wake."

"Is that just you or is this the general way of things." I asked.

"Yer, eet's all over loik thut. You ask onyone, yer comes, dost thou beet, en goss. Way ev a few bargies en faytes – eets normal loik. Theer's a fayte on at market this Saturday, effen yer interested, loik. One of our lads is a praize boxer so way're o going to egg 'im on. Thah's a cup en o fer the winner... en praize monney. Eet's a big thing 'ere int' Potteries."

"Yes, maybe." really just brushing this invitation aside and continued. "Doesn't anyone check the number of pieces you produce? Isn't there a set amount that has to be produced every day or week?"

"Orr, dunno abite thut. Na-one checks. Way jest gets peeyed aych wayk. Thut's all ah nahs. Ah mayt go in on Wednesday en di o'er 'ours to cetch up though."

So, there seemed to be only the loosest daily or weekly supervision of the workpeople, in their separate "shops", and working by "piece-work", the workers produced as much as they wanted, when they wanted. The weekly production of each worker was not scanned as it was in a cotton mill. Hundreds of workpeople never did a day's work for the first two days of the week. Drinking or pure idleness were seen and winked at by the employers. It was never considered that, if a week's work had to be done in four days, it must be scamped to a great extent. If a man worked for these four days until 10 o'clock at night, or began at 4 or 5am, this did not concern the "master". There was loss, of course, in the use of coal for these extra hours, but this didn't disturb any sense of economy, as it wasn't monitored A man might begin to do his work on Wednesday morning, half asleep or half drunk, after two or three days' debauch, and nothing would be said apart from some jibe or other. It was a sort of pawn shop method of doing business – pawn something one week and take it out another, when you need it. So it was with business, have a slack week, then make up for it the next. Most of the pot owners shied clear of introducing machinery – they couldn't anyway. These pot-banks had been built up in a ramshackle way, built round hovels and under archways, side by side with another. There was very little space and tortuous ways of getting into them.

Jimmy continued as I bandaged his wounds. "'Cos, ef the Master should paye us a visit, way all looks as ef way're warking 'ard. Gee a kick to the drunks folling aslayp at theer teebles. Somwon 'll whistle ef they say the Master coming en way put on a show, all quayet loik. 'E nivver says onything onyways - not normally onyways – jest passes through wi' is 'ands tucked, at the bek, onder his tailcoat. Donna git may wrung – way dunna want te come te 'is attention. Ah maynes, 'es the Master. Ef ah'm thron aht, ah'll nivver get a riference fer owt else. Ah toffs mar cap te 'im en nay uther."

I gleaned from this that the master wasn't looking at anything in particular and, in consequence, saw nothing. He didn't notice the drunkards at their work tables or notice how many workers were there at a particular time.

It would have been better if there were machinery in the Potteries, to necessitate discipline. This would also have promoted cost calculation, which seemed to be woefully deficient in the Potteries. The workers lived like children, without any calculating forecast of their work or its result. The great co-operative societies would never have risen to such immense and fruitful development but for the calculating induced by the use of machinery. Trades unions had infiltrated the Potteries but they were haphazard and surrounded by suspicion. Even those who relied on the unions for protection, looked at them with misgiving and thought of them as 'poachers' – something else you had to pay for!

I recalled speaking to another of my patients, Alice, who lived in a hovel, barely able to support herself and had to stop work for the time being owing to her painfully cracked fingers caused by the lead exuding from the paints used. As she couldn't work, she had no money coming in and was relying on friends and neighbours for a little bit of food. I spoke to her about possibly joining a trade union.

"Don't you think a trade union would be able to help you and your colleagues? They'd be able to fight for your rights and protect you – fight for a better way of working – look into the possibility of someone being able to eliminate the toxins in the paint and also provide payment to you when you're too ill to work.?"

"Ah dunno abite thut, duckie. Ah'm a Methodist en way Methodists think theer the divil's wark. Ah conna go agin the church, now cod ah? They nahs best, duckie. Ah'm a good Methodist, may. Ah conna write much but ah con rayd Bable."

Yes, I remember thinking to myself – the whole area is under the Methodist blanket and, even though someone doesn't class themselves as such, they will have attended Sunday schools and been indoctrinated and, therefore, distrustful of all associations which were condemned by religious people. Even those who did not regularly attend places of worship would be seen on the Sabbath 'in their Sunday best', except for those seen as a lower class of people, the plate-makers and slip-makers, who could not afford Sunday best.

....

One good thing, though, that came out of the general strike, was that pay-cuts could no longer be implemented and workers learnt from this that, by their efforts and through their strike they had gained at least a partial victory, a powerful impetus was given towards the creation of trade unions.

After the Chartists riots in 1842 the local force was replaced by a body of country police and, by 1851 this comprised a superintendent, an inspector and 20 men.

Also, on 7 November 1842, the Miners' Association of Great Britain and Ireland was formally established at Wakefield.

At a North Staffs coal trade meeting in December, it was decided to tolerate the existence of the Miners' Association in the coalfield.

In December 1843 the Shelton miners, many of them not in the union, went on strike and won a wage increase.

Even after all this it was still the general feeling in Parliament, at the time, that, if the working classes were given the vote, the monarchy could not survive. The lower classes, once given supreme power, through ignorance, wouldn't know what to do with it, and would not be likely to respect the institution of property. They believed the lower classes wished for monopoly of land and machinery and ownership to cease, leading to plunder of every man in the kingdom who had a roof over his head. Military rule would be necessitated, and the nation would never again see the likes of the liberty, wealth, knowledge and arts the country had produced. All the nations which envied our greatness would insult our downfall.

In March 1860 arguments ensued in Parliament again for a Reform Act. I followed this avidly in the newspaper reports. Lord Palmerston, the Prime Minister, was opposed to parliamentary reform. Again, he argued that unions were exciting the working classes. The direct consequence would be an increased cry for the ballot and the introduction of men into the House of Commons. Once trade unionists had the vote they would demand the reduction of the working day to eight hours. Benjamin Disraeli (Conservative) argued that the enfranchisement of 203,000 people would mean these people would cast their votes as one body and power would be conferred to the lower class. However, William Gladstone, the Chancellor of the Exchequer, and who had been a member of the Conservative Party, and had originally opposed parliamentary reform, had changed his mind following a tour of the cotton district, and had been favourably impressed by working-class qualities. He became convinced that large numbers of working-class men could be trusted to exercise the franchise responsibly.

However, Lord Palmerston died in July 1865 and Earl Russell became Prime Minister. On 12 March 1866 William Gladstone introduced the government's new Reform Bill with the vote going to occupiers of property in the boroughs worth £7 in rent a year. So, probably about one in four men would have been able to vote, instead of the existing one in five. Gladstone had calculated that, while increasing the number of working-class voters, it would still have left them a minority of the total electorate.

Gladstone argued that the wages of a man occupying such a house would be a little under 26s a week. That sum would certainly be unobtainable by the peasantry, and by mere labourers, but is generally obtainable by artisans and skilled labourers. There was argument against this too. Robert Lowe brought into account the possibility of wage rises and rental increases – which would lead, sooner or later, to the number of working classes allowed to vote, being in majority. He had gone on to say that, if you want ignorance, drunkenness, impulsive unreflecting and violent people getting the vote, look no further than those living in small houses. This class of people getting the majority vote, would lead to an increase of corruption, intimidation and disorder. With this argument, Russell's government found it impossible to get the bill passed by the House of Commons and Russell resigned on 19th June 1866.

As a response to this, the Reform League organised a great street procession and meeting of 30,000 strong in support of the popular demand for household suffrage. The London press, for days after the procession, had marched through the principal street of the fashionable West End, teemed with half-frightened references to, its military aspects, good marching, admirable order, well closed column and complete discipline."

Lord Russell retired in 1867 and Gladstone became leader of the Liberal Party. He continued his attempts to increase the number of people who could vote. Edward Smith-Stanley, leading the Conservative Party, was now sympathetic to the idea. Disraeli, the new leader of the House of Commons, stepped in at this point, fearing that voters would run to the Liberal Party, and changed tactics. He reasoned that, if the Conservatives could pilot a reform bill through Parliament, they might gain politically as the newly enfranchised in the boroughs might well vote Conservative out of gratitude. At the same time they could make sure the bill had the necessary precautions to preserve aristocratic power in the counties. He proposed a new Reform Act in March 1867. Fewer working class males would get the vote and, in addition, university graduates, members of the learned professions and those with £50 savings were to have extra votes.

On 21st March 1867 Gladstone made a two hour speech in the House of Commons, exposing, in detail, the inconsistencies of the bill, proposing an amendment which would allow a tenant to vote whether or not he paid his own rates. Forty-three members of his own party voted with the Conservatives and the amendment was defeated. Gladstone was so angry that apparently he contemplated retirement to the backbench.

I began to relate this to Theresa May's party, trying to get Brexit through, in 2016/19, as 17.4 million people had voted to leave the EU. So many of her own party were against her and, although she got a very slim backing to remain as Prime Minister, her Brexit plan was defeated over and over, mainly because she had so many remainers in her party, who were actually getting EU ministers to oppose her in any way they could. She was also hampered by Jeremy Corbyn, for Labour, putting the spoke in time and time again; firstly agreeing to accept her deal, then when it came to the vote, declining to back her, requesting a second referendum; then requesting a 'no deal' being taken off the table, when a 'no deal' was the only deal that would take us forward, even though a 'no deal' had been rejected in one of the votes anyway. In fact, things were so grim that Theresa May was forced to agree to resign as soon the UK had left the EU, whether this was with a deal or not. (In fact, she resigned beforehand, leaving the contenders to debate amongst themselves who was to become the leader of the Conservative party). No-one wanted her Chequers Plan because it basically meant that Northern Ireland would have to have a hard customs border with Southern Ireland and also it would leave the UK as puppets to the EU – i.e. having to obey any EU laws, but not be allowed any say in the making of these laws. Everything was up in the air, with Theresa May making her way back to Brussels again and again in a vain attempt to get changes made to her deal, as the EU were not prepared to agree to any changes. In the end, the feeling was that Theresa May never wanted her deal to go through anyway and she was, initially, herself, a remainer, plus the fact the she insisted on wearing red, the Labour colour, which infuriated many staunch Tories. She even has a wax model of her in Madam Tussaud's, wearing red!. Margaret Thatcher, no matter how disliked in the end, would never have been seen wearing red.

Everyone was up in arms, Remainers and Brexiteers, and totally left bewildered as to who to vote for. The UK was on the brink of a constitutional crisis. The Wetherspoon's letters in their magazine, written by Professor Robert Tombs, Historian and Author, and Sir Noel Malcolm, Senior research fellow at All Souls College Oxford, actually stated that, on the strength of research older, poorer or less educated people were more likely to have voted for Brexit'. Also, Remainer and former MP Matthew Parris stated that, for him, Brexit means 'trusting the people. "I don't", he wrote, "Never have and never will". He saw his job as 'curbing the instincs of the mob'. The enlightened elite must govern by subterfuge, if necessary. That, I felt, was such a backward step. The fight by the Chartists to get their People's Charter through Parliament over 170 years ago, to get the vote for everyone, was refused time and time again, as the elitist aristocrats believed the populace too uneducated to be given the vote in the first place. They believed wholeheartedly that, if they were, they wouldn't know what to do with it, and the years taken to built up Great Britain into a great nation, would be lost to civil war and anarchy forever. So, nothing had changed in 170 years - the elite still thought the populace know nothing and are not to be trusted, no matter how educated they are and apprised as to what is happening in politics, having access to all arguments and manifestos via their computers and smartphones. The 17.4 million people who voted for Brexit, were basically inept white, elderly, uneducated persons, who should have their ability to vote removed from them. They want us to return to pre-1867.

Back in 1867, however, some members of the aristocracy declared that the people should not be heard in the councils of the nation – which was a very dangerous and criminal thing. The general populace had fought so vehemently for their rights and members of the Reform League were still advocating the need for universal suffrage. There was a large rally in Birmingham. The landlords, army and navy lords and law lords, who looked eagerly for a share of taxes for themselves and their dependants, would never let the people's noses from the grindstone, if they could help it. But the people had the power in their hands. They had to show they were prepared to burst open the doors of the House of Commons should they be kept persistently closed against them.

On 18th April 1867 the Reform League's executive council met in London and unanimously condemned Disraeli's Bill and reaffirmed their commitment to "a vote for a man, because he is a man". A national demonstration was called in Hyde Park – this took place on 6th May. The Home Secretary, Spencer Walpole, denounced any such meeting as illegal and warned that any people attending this meeting would be at their peril. The Government arranged for troops of Hussars to be deployed in the park and thousands of special constables were sworn in. However, after seeing the thousands of demonstrators that turned up – anything between 20,000 to 500,000, according to what paper I read, it was decided to back down. Bradlaugh commented that the reformers who had been killed at Peterloo were now at last victorious. Following this, Walpole resigned.

On 20th May Disraeli accepted an amendment from Grosvenor Hodgkinson, which added nearly half a million voters to the electoral rolls, therefore doubling the effect of the bill.

The 1867 Reform Act gave the vote to every male householder living in a borough constituency. Male lodgers paying £10 for unfurnished rooms were also granted the vote. This gave the vote to about 1,500,000 men. A more even distribution of MPs was agreed with boroughs of less than 10,000 inhabitants losing an MP. The forty-five seats left available were distributed by giving fifteen to towns which had never had an MP; giving one extra seat to some larger towns, i.e. Liverpool, Manchester, Birmingham and Leeds; creating a seat for the University of London; and giving twenty-five seats to counties whose population had increased since 1832.

Of course, women weren't given the vote yet (unless, of course, they were owners of property), although there were great suffrage movements taking place to obtain this. In fact, there was actually some debate against, as most women at the time were either not interested or did not feel capable of going against their domineering husbands, and said they did not want women's suffrage. Most lower class women had not even had much of schooling, except Sunday school, and could not read or write. They would sign their name on any document, such as a marriage certificate, with a cross – X.

Yes, I remember going back in my own family history and getting certificates copied, to see that my great grandmother had signed a X for her signature, on a birth certificate.

CHAPTER 4 – SCHOOL

I tried my best to keep John warm, lighting a fire, putting a clay hot water bottle in with him and massaging his feet. I also remembered to open a window slightly. Florence Nightingale would have been proud of me. It was one of her commandments that there should be adequate ventilation in a sick person's room, not just from an open door, but from an open window, to let fresh air in. This of course, was bearing in mind that the window didn't open onto a pig sty or heap of effluent.

John was awake at last. "Come on John. Let's see if we can get you off that horribly hard door you're lying on and change the bedding." I tried to support his back and he attempted to swing his legs off the bed but it was too much of an effort for him. He was aching. "Ah canna, Jane. Ah'm just say brittle." I felt really sorry for him. What could I do? I didn't want to give him more morphine. Aspirin hadn't been invented yet – ah, but I knew the basic ingredient came from the bark of the willow tree. It had been used over the centuries for a home cure for pain. During my time as nurse in the area, I'd come across people who knew the old ways. Mrs Green was one of them. She was the midwife at Bagnall. She lived in one of the cottages past the stone quarry by the Almshead Road. Both of us went round together sometimes when a baby was coming. I learnt a lot from her. Plus my memories of "Call the Midwife" came in handy, knowing what to do with breach births and the like. I loved that series – set in Poplar, London and covering quite a few decades of the early to mid 20th century. Mrs Green was a character. She used to make wine. Elderberry, potato, all sorts. She also used to distil whisky. She had to bury it on the common in case she got caught. Anyway, she'd shown me how to make a pain-reliever from the willow tree, made into a simple herbal tea. The white willow was the best as it contains more of the acid than the other varieties of willow. John was weak but his pulse was stable now. I decided to get one of the neighbours to keep an eye on him and go in search of my willow tree. It would be hard work and tedious but John needed any help I could give him.

What you get from the willow bark is the raw material from which acetylsalicylic acid is made, the main ingredient of aspirin. You have to be careful with it and make sure it isn't too concentrated, as then it could be dangerous and cause stomach-bleeding. Mrs Green had used it for years with no ill affects whatsoever. After finding the tree, she'd cut a square from the bark. There is an outer bark and an inner bark and it's the inner bark that is used, so you need to cut deep. You need the bark to come off in one piece. Some of the inner bark is white and some pinkish in colour. It's the pinkish bark that is needed. Once you have your square, about as big as your palm, cut off the pinkish bark. When home you proceed to make the tea by filtering it through muslin cloth, then wrapping it up like a tea bag. Throw this tea bag into a pot of boiling water. Stir it periodically, and keep an eye on the colour of the water. It will slowly begin to take on a deep reddish-brown colour, almost like the colour of blood. Now you just have to filter out any remaining solids using a tea-strainer. You need to strain it again through muslin cloth. Once it has stopped dripping, squeeze the muslin to get the liquid out, so that it drips into a mug. Once all the liquid has been squeezed out, keep filtering until all the liquid has been filtered into a mug. After about 20 minutes, the tea should be ready. You're not to overcook it or you will burn the medicine out of it. Once it is done boiling, let it steep a few minutes. Just add some sugar (if required) and drink. It's not strong enough for real pain but it helps.

"Whut'r yer friggling wi?" John asked rather hoarsely.

"Just something to help with your pain." So, I'd made the infusion and presented it to John. "Here John, sip this. You should begin to feel a bit better in a while." I got behind him so he could rest against me to take the potion.

"Eet's owe rate, Jane. Thank 'ee".

It was so relieving to hear John actually able to talk. I'd thought I'd lost him. John hadn't really lost his strong Potteries dialect, even after all these years, but then we'd been apart from each other for so long. If we'd stayed together, maybe my own way of speaking would have rubbed off onto him, but I didn't really mind. It was part of his character.

"Ah dunna want te mither yer, but cosna git a message te William Meigh playse thut ah canna wark. Tell 'im ah'll bay on mar fayt agin sooen."

"It's OK John, don't worry. I've already sent one of the neighbour's lads to Ash Hall. They know all about the flooding at the pit and that you were taken ill going down the mine, trying your best to save Alfred."

64

"'Anna 'eerd onythin' abite Alfred, Jane? 'As evera one bin wi' a message?"

"Not yet, love. I still have hopes. I've been with you all the time, so I don't know what's happening there. If they've managed to get him out, we'll soon hear, one way or another."

John put his hand on mine, which was resting on his shoulder. "'Dunna fayre, Jane. Whut'll bay will bay. Wey con onnly 'ope."

It's then I realised that I'd been so caught up with John that I hadn't given a thought to Alfred's wife and children. Kate would be worried out of her life. They had two little children, Mary Annie, who was 7, and little William, who was only 1. I'd have to see if I could get a message to her, let her know that John was improving slowly, though still in a lot of pain.

I took the mug away from John and laid him softly back down onto the bed.

"Yer raight, thus bed's as 'ard as a dooer." To which we both laughed, but then I started to sob again. It was more a sob of relief than anything else. That was my John, cracking a joke at the worst of times.

"'Hay, lass, dunna wereet yersen so."

"I know, it's just so good to have you back in the land of the living. I still love you John, no matter what has happened over the years."

"Ay, way'll say, Jane. Ah knahs. Ah loves yer too, especially o yer've don fer may. Yer've saved mar loif! Ah wodna bay 'ere wi'ite you, Jane. Thut's fer sure."

I bent over and kissed him on the forehead.

"'As it 'appens, ah'm beginnin' te fayl a mite better. Mebbee ah con tray agin te git missen oop."

"OK, if you think you're up to it, I'll give you a hand. There you go." I supported him as he made a very tentative step to the rocking chair and plonked down heavily in it. "Here, let's put the blanket around you to keep you warm, while I get rid of this disgusting door and remake the bed for you.

"Yer, gooed redance – ah wanna com knockin' on you agin, dooer, nay fayer, yer've don yer duty, now bay off wi' yer."

"That's it, John. Give it a good telling off."

While John was there, I made him some soup with bread. "Thank 'ee, Jane. Ah cod ate a man uff 'is 'orse ent' saddle en o." I realised I was really hungry too. It hadn't occurred to me before that I hadn't had anything to eat since the disaster. I hadn't thought of food as I was too worried about John to realise I was quite famished.

I helped John back to bed afterwards and went to do the washing up. There was no running water, so water had to be brought in a bucket from the well in Washerwall and heated up on the range. Luckily John had got me one of the better ranges that had a water-heating tank attached to it. You had to keep it filled up and the range on but you could have hot water just by opening a tap on this tank and putting a bucket underneath to catch the hot water.

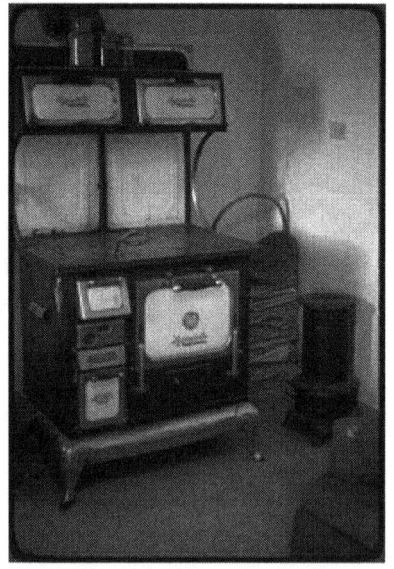

The Sherwins keep the well clean and they are very particular. They have a cottage right by the well. They won't let children play on the green around it and keep the grass cut short. They charge a shilling a year to draw water from the well. Mr Sherwin is known as 'peg leg' because he only has the one leg.

The water from the well is the best in the area and they take wooden barrels by cart to Hanley and sell their water by the bucketful. It never runs dry like other wells. If you go on a real hot day in summer and get a cup of water from that well, it is like drinking fresh snow. The farmer's wives, when they are making butter, need sixteen buckets of water. They put a bit of carrot in the water to give the butter a good colour – it made it look yellow and rich. Another part of the Sherwin family have a farm at the corner of Draw-Well Lane. He has a pony and trap that he would hire out, which was handy.

Dr Knight, from Bucknall, comes each week, wearing his top hat, to drink from the well and to fill his large glass bottles to mix his medicines for his patients in Bucknall and Werrington.

Looking out of the kitchen window I saw a couple of young lads playing marbles in the street, or 'chuck i' th 'ole', as they called it. They were not like the marbles I played with in my youth, which were glass with coloured cats' eye shapes in the centre. I could see, what they called, a 'rinker', a larger black marble with white spots, the king of marbles in an era when all children played the game. I heard them calling out 'crogs, no peys', meaning the marble is shifted without forfeit, and 'fogger' denoting the first in the game. One of them produced a glassey (a marble made of glass) and there were also stonies, taws and alleys.

I opened the door and called out to them. They were John Sherwin, who lived at No. 30 and Enoch Hewitt, who lived at No.29. They were both 8 years old. "John, Enoch, can you take a message for me. It's a long trek to 34 Bucknall Old Road. There's a farthing in it each for you. Just tell Mrs Wood that her father-in-law is recovering slowly and ask if she's heard any news about her husband. Now, can you remember that?"

"Olraight," John answered, repeated my message then both scarpered off down the road.

....
Thinking of their journey, I imagined their route but then my imagination took a turn to the general area. The tree tops, either side of the Werrington Road, touched and formed arches from Brookhouse Farm to Four Lanes End. In summer it was like walking in a green cathedral. Squirrels leaped from branch to branch and seemed to keep you company. A raised voice at the bridge could be heard more than half a mile up the hill.

The stream cooled the silver milk churns at Little Brookhouse Farm and flowed over sandstone and bubbles toward the marsh where marigolds lifted their yellow cups to sun and rain. It was here that oxbows formed at Bucknall Sands as it spread over the lower ground and passed Lily Dale and Nellie Dale and the coal mining spoil..... where my poor Alfred would be, probably dead or breathing his last breath. I found myself wringing my hands and tears forming and that hallucination came to the fore of John and me floating in the inky-black ocean, not able to see or hear anything, with my screams echoing around me. A cold shiver went down my spine. NO, I didn't want to think too hard about this scene, so I forced myself to continue my imaginary walk, which turned eventually to the hamlet of The Green, where the ducks from the cottages swam the stream before it went on to turn two of the Bucknall mills on its way to join the River Trent.

I started day-dreaming, while looking out of the kitchen window, thinking about people in our little hamlet. They were good children around here. Doing their bit just to earn a farthing or two. They'd walk from Washwell Lane (as it was called on those days) to Moorville Hall, where there's a big wood. They'd pick bilberries at 5 o'clock in the morning and sell them to the womenfolk in the houses. They also got blackberries when they were in season. The money they collected meant they could buy clothes as their parents were so hard up. They'd also fetch buckets of water from a stream on the moor to sell to folk. They'd pull it on a little wooden cart with a rope attached. Most families kept a pig or two and the womenfolk would do laundry or sewing to get a bob or two. Most of the men in Washerwell were colliers. Out of 27 homesteads in 1861, 18 worked in the mines, 1 carter, 1 stonemason, 1 butcher and son, 6 farmers, 1 in the potteries, 1 labourer, 1 agricultural labourer, 1 blacksmith, 2 grocers' assistants and 1 gardener. The miners would set of at 5am to walk up Washwall Lane to work. Nobody needed clocks or watches – you knew what time it was when you heard the miners' clogs go up and down the lane. Of course, when the miners were working, the wives had money, and would boast about how much they had in their little tin boxes.

In summer time, when the miners couldn't sell the coal, they used to go to Cheshire to get any work they could, mowing - by hand with a scythe as there was no machinery in those days, leaving their families at home and stay and lodge in Cheshire.

The women all hung their washing on a piece of land near to the well. They got real nasty if a woman got her washing out regularly before the others. I'd seen a women cut someone else's clothes line and she came back later to find her washing lying in the mud. They weren't all friendly and nice, only in times of trouble.

I would sometimes watch in fascination as the ladies at Bleach House, in Washerwall, stretched out their washed and bleached fabrics, by the well, onto poles, that they called tenterhooks, leaving them out to dry.

Isaacs Bettaney lived in Washwell Lane. He was born in 1807. He was a farmer labourer but built himself up and built all the stone walls down this road and round these fields. He built them from Four Lane End to the last cottage at the bottom of Washwell Lane. He moved houses, first living at No 19, then at No 9, then No. 1. Bettaneys owned most of the houses in the village. Roggin Row belonged to them at one time and Little Widow Farm. His son, Thomas, was born in 1850 and, when he was older, worked as a collier, and lived at No. 1 Washwell Lane.

Old Tommy Profitt owned the stone quarry right at the top of the common. It was called The Peak. He lived at No. 32 Washwell Lane and was born in 1821. He had a son, also called Tommy, born 1855. They carted the stone to the Potteries. Either it was ground up for sand to make bricks, or the potters had it. The road he had to use along Washerwall was only a track. In winter it was knee deep in mud. When they were not busy, they would send a loaded cart to drop great lumps of stone in the sludge to make the road. All of their carts and everybody else's would crush over it all winter. When summer came, their men would dig it up, sieve it, cart it to the Potteries and sell it for making saggars. They filled the holes up with another load of stone the next winter. Old Tommy

Profitt's wife used to wear a great big hat, it had embroidery of birds and flowers on it. She used to draw the sand money every Saturday and they would both get drunk. They'd come down the lane and be so sozzled she'd be staggering along with her hat tipped over one eye.

Mr Proffitt used to preach at the old chapel in the lane. Mrs Proffitt used to go to chapel, every Sunday, when Tommy was a baby. She'd have him in her arms and used to take him with her for the service at night. If he started squawking, she'd unfasten her blouse, let it flop out and give him a suck, in chapel! I remembered there was an outcry in 2019 about women suckling their young in public and whether or not it should be allowed. I don't remember what the outcome was though.

At farmers' market time, I used to see herds of cattle and sheep being driven along Ash Bank to the auctions at Leek, about six miles away. Young kids would be herding the cattle. It took them about 2½ to 3 hours normally. It was good to take a break and see the horse fairs at Leek, just camp out somewhere and walk home the next day.

I felt sorry for the poor children, and they were poor. Even when Christmas came, all they had was an orange and apple as a treat. They had no overcoats in winter, nothing to keep them warm, especially the poorer families in Bucknall. If it was wet they would get an old coal sack, split up one side to put over their heads. They would wrap sacks around their leg, tied round with string to keep them warm and dry. If they were lucky, they had clogs for shoes. Winters here could be wild in Werrington, with gales and gusting winds, that blew everything around that wasn't tied down and we had snow every couple of days through January and sometimes snow even into April.

If anyone had anything substantial to eat, it was always the father. He'd get beef every Sunday, while the children just had the gravy. The father had a bacon breakfast every morning before going to work. His wife would have to make a fire up especially. The kiddies just had to make do with bread and jam. Of course, there was no toothpaste as such, many used charcoal to clean their teeth, if they did at all, so you'd see many adults with bad teeth, or gaps where teeth had fallen out, due to their bad diet.

There had been the Sunday schools, where children were taught bible lessons and little classrooms run by women, to teach kiddies until they could go out to get a job at 7 or 8 years old. There had also been Ragged Schools then, the only possibility of education for those families who had been turned away from other charitable or church schools and whose parents couldn't pay for their children to learn. Children who went to Ragged Schools tended to be poor and commonly came from families where parents were abusive or drunks. Some pupils were orphaned and some pupils' parents were in prison so they had taken to sleeping on the streets. The Ragged Schools gave free meals and clothing to their pupils and taught them a trade such as shoemaking or domestic skills. There, they were washed and given clothes to wear during the day, but these clothes were taken off them at the end of each school day as they knew that the parents would immediately whip the clothes of the kiddies backs and sell them.

There were, of course, pay-schools, but most of the parents in the Potteries and thereabouts could not afford to put their children into school, and they needed the little money that the children brought in from their work in the factories.

The Factory Act of 1833, had imposed a duty on employers to provide half-time education for employees under 13. In practice, the Act was easily ignored.

However, things had gradually started to change.

In 1846 the government began to help pay for teacher training too, which would serve to help more teachers get the training they needed ,successfully, to teach this generation of young people who were, one day, to lead the country to new heights.

Things had changed dramatically by 1870 with the introduction of the 1870 Education Act. Elected school boards could levy a local rate to build new schools, providing education up to the age of 10. In 1880 the provision of elementary schooling for both sexes was made compulsory, and the age raised to 13. However, by 1870 there was growing pressure for provision of schools in areas where none existed. There was a conflict of opinion over whether the state should pay for schools run by the church. The leading industrialists had realised that education was necessary to lead Britain in its industrial progress and maintain its lead in manufacture. Britain was going through an amazing, prosperous period of industrialisation and the British Empire was growing. There was a serious need to educate all the British people to help drive Britain forward and be able to show off its citizens to the world. These young people were the future of Great Britain, the then capital of the world. The days were gone in which it was acceptable to worry that, by letting poorer children go to school to learn, they would become unhappy with their social standing.

Every child was to be given a place at school and school buildings had to be of a reasonable quality. Head teachers now had to be qualified too. Schools throughout the nation were inspected and checked to make sure that the education they were offering met the new standards. New rules now meant that school boards could make school compulsory for children between five and ten years old and later thirteen.

Over the next ten years, new schools were set up in areas, where there had been none before, making education accessible for everyone. School boards were set up to manage and build these.

So the bill was passed, which allowed voluntary schools to carry on unchanged, but established a system of 'school boards' to build and manage schools in areas where they were needed. These boards were locally elected bodies, drawing their funding from the local rates. However, this act still didn't make education compulsory. The 1876 Royal Commission on the Factory Acts recommended that education be made compulsory in order to stop the abusive conduct of factory owners by taking children off the streets, into their factories, to pay them pennies for 16 hours work a day – a brilliant way to enhance the koffers of the already rich. Children were thought nothing of - they were just a way of getting cheap labour. It wasn't until 1880 that a further Education Act finally made school attendance compulsory between the ages of five and ten, though still only got 82% attendance. Truancy was a problem, due to the fact that parents could not afford to give up income earned by their children.

So, John Sherwin and Enoch Hewitt were just playing hooky.

Of course, John and Enoch's school would have been a lot better than when Victoria first came to the throne, but I bet they didn't realise this! When Victoria first came to the throne a school then would have been cold in winter as there may not have been a fire to heat your room or school hall. If there was, you may have been sat so far away that the warmth didn't reach you! Having most probably walked to school, you might spend much of your time in wet, cold clothes from your journey in, depending on the time of year and you would certainly be tired – sometimes, children would have to walk a long way to school! When you got there, you would fully expect to be inspected by your teacher and would have to be smartly turned out. Respect for your teacher was very important and you would bow or curtsy to them during registration.

Lessons would be in the three 'R's: Reading, wRiting and aRithmetic. Sometimes, schools would teach geography, history and 'drill', the Victorian equivalent of PE. You probably wouldn't have had your own books; instead, they would be shared among the whole class and kept by the teacher on his or her desk, which would be at the front of the room. You would have a slate and chalk to write on. Depending on which school you went to, you may or may not have a break time! During lessons, you would be expected to pay attention and work to a high standard. If the child made a mistake, such as a wrong spelling, the child would be requested to repeatedly write out the correct misspelling. Writing with your left hand was a no-no – the child would have his left hand tied behind his back to prevent him using it to write. Punishments would either be painful or humiliating and might be either a sharp rap across the knuckles with a cane or being sent to the corner to wear the dunce's cap – often with your face to the wall in shame. If you accidentally fell asleep in class, you could expect to receive a nasty snap of the master's ruler or perhaps even being woken up with some very cold water!

However, Victoria had a significant influence on education and, towards the end of the century, education was a very different animal to what it had been. Although there was still a huge difference between schools then and now, significant improvements had taken place in the space of fifty years. Many of the town schools even had libraries as well as pianos. As well as the three 'R's, subjects studied might include sport such as cricket, plus needlework, drawing and craft work, map drawing, geography, history, religion, gardening and music. Some schools had also begun to have special rooms for science and cookery. Schools were giving awards and prizes to encourage progress and hard work. Pupils were being closely monitored and a Queen Victoria Medal might be awarded to pupils with outstanding attendance in recognition of the importance of school and a pupil's commitment. A very different story to the beginning of the century education. Opportunity to learn and progress was greater than ever...for everyone.

Still, who could beat a game of marbles on a nice sunny day rather than being stuck in a room and having to concentrate on every word the teacher said, when the sun is making you feel drowsy. Anyway, I was glad they were there, so they could take my message to Albert's wife.

CHAPTER 5 – WERRINGTON

I did my best at Christmas, making paper chains out of old newspapers and anything colourful I could find, and cut down a little fir tree, put it into a bucket filled with earth and made little fancy bows from ribbon to tie to each branch, with a little doll on top that I'd added white fabric wings to. No-one had ever seen the like, and all the local kiddies came to see it. Stoke tried its best, even though there was no electricity for fairy lights. They got a fir tree each year and decorated it as best they could. Of course, we all read about Queen Victoria and her Christmas tree. Prince Albert was presented with a tree in 1841 and installed it and decorated it at Windsor Castle. It had long been a German tradition to have Christmas trees. It was decorated beautifully. On the branches they hung little nets made from cut-out coloured paper. Every net was filled with goodies and golden apples and walnuts hung down as if they grew there and they tied little candles, red, white and blue, to the different boughs. High on the summit of the tree was fixed a tinsel star.

．．．．．．．

John and I had lived in our little two-bed stone cottage, in the hamlet of Washerwall, that is until John moved out. He went to live at the gatehouse at the rear of Ash Hall, in Brookhouse Road. Washerwall is a nice community with no pub, thank goodness. Someone had tried to build a pub but had run out of money. I'd seen enough of the good-for-nothing drunkards pouring out of the pubs.

All the houses in Washerwall were built of stone. There is a little grocer's shop at No. 28 Washerwall, owned by Caroline Bloor and someone actually tried to open a fish and chip shop, but it failed. My cottage is in a row of four, near the Common end (just before where Moorland Aveue is now). At the other end is a little shop called Mifflin's. There's also a shop called Dales in the middle of the row of cottages. I was lucky that John had put the outside toilet in for us, as the other cottages had to share two toilets between them, that were on the other side of the road. One was a 'flush type' but with no running water, so they still had to take a bucket of water with them to flush out the toilets.

I lime-wash ours every year. It has a wooden seat. I remember having an outside toilet when I was growing up, in London. It had a wooden seat too and one time it got a crack in it. I hadn't realised and ooh it did pinch me. Obviously we got a new one. Still, these outside toilets are darned awkward to keep clean. Any living, crawling insect will get in. You'd be sitting there then notice out of the corner of your eye something dangling down from the ceiling – a great big spider. It's worse in winter as most lavatory doors have cracks in them. The doors are short and about six inches off the floor, allowing the winter wind to blow in. There's a window high on the back wall with a couple of bricks knocked out and no glass, so just a hole. In winter, the wind just blows right through. In summer, the toilets stink and swarm with flies. I put disinfectant down and around the floor, so do my best, and keep old newspapers to use, as toilet paper had not been produced yet.

John had done the best with ours and had built a piped runway into a covered sewerage pit. He'd also put a new door on. He couldn't install running water though, even though the well was just over the way, as it is a limited supply and we have to pay for it, so we got, and I still get, buckets of water from another brook, or Coffin Well to swill it down.

Mr Shenton and someone else, probably Mr Wilshaw, do the night soiling. They go all over the place collecting muck. They get it out of the closets to spread on the fields, in the mistaken belief that it will provide manure for plants. They collect it from Bucknall Fever Hospital too. The paper is the worst as, if it is windy, this dirty, soiled paper blows about off the fields. I remember they told me a story once about going to Bryan Street in Hanley. There are many Irish, who came over, following the Irish potato famine, and stayed. It had been night-time and there was a wedding going on. There was only one room, which they had to pass through to empty the closet in the back yard. The place was teaming with folk, so they kept going in backward and forwards with buckets full, and every time they passed through the room, these Irish folk gave them a cup of whisky. Nobody seemed bothered at all and they never seemed to notice the stink! Oh well, it's what you get used to. I remembered going to Venice for the first time, in the 1970s and the stink really hit you but, after a couple of days, you didn't notice it.

There are actually two quarries in Washerwall, one of which is for building stone, owned by Old Tommy Profitt, and the other for sand. The sand is obtained by crushing a fine stone superimposed on the millstone grit and is of such excellent quality that it is in great demand in the Potteries for 'placing' ware. The Sherratts own this quarry. They are a big family. Simon Sherratt once lived at No. 32 Washerwall. He is the father of Emma Sherratt.. William Sherratt lives at No. 15 Werrington. Charles Sherratt lives at Moss House, Washerwall – he is a sand dealer.

We had our own little Methodist church, just by the quarry but in 1860 Emma Sherratt bought it and had it as a house. She paid for it all in silver threepenny bits, so I heard. She must have been saving them for years, from her wages. This Emma Sherratt was hard as nails – she works in the sand quarry in Washerwall, with her brother, Charlie, working all hours, grinding sand. At night she breaks the stone ready to grind into sand the next day. What a job! But she never complains – just gets on with it. I think she must wrap her hands in old cloths, but I bet they are still covered in callouses. They have a gin rig with a horse that goes round and round and crushes it. The sand is then carted to the towns for making into pots. Of course, both quarries in 21st century have been built on with housing.

Coal is sixpence a hundred-weight. She fetches coal from a foot rail on the common for anybody in the lane who wants it. She takes a wheelbarrow and trundles a bag of coal for threepence. She also fetches water for Sherwins and Bettanys right at the top of the lane. She carries the water from both wells, wearing a yoke over her shoulders with two buckets for the spring drinking water – washing water she takes in a drum. She has a sort of dolly tub on wheels, which she fills using a bucket at Coffin Well, covers the top with a sack bag, puts on a harness of straps, as you would do to a horse, and just pulls it! Washing day she carts for sixpence a day. Coffin Well was a long stone well, presumably named as it resembled a coffin.

The Forresters live at Cabin Croft, just on the edge of the Common. It is a thatched cottage. Ralph Forrester has a large orchard at the back of his farm. His wife sells all the fruit off the trees and the eggs and cream she sells to a place next to the Trumpet public house in Hanley. So, when I need eggs and milk or fruit, I take a trail up to the cottage.

There are two other industries in Werrington - weaving is carried on in the cottages opposite the Windmill Inn and in the stable of the Home Office School farm, which was built in 1752. The materials used are sacking and gingham. Daniel Hassell, master weaver, of Foxearth, was still there in 1852. He was about 60 then, so I suppose he's no longer with us. Nail-making is the other industry. These are family industries, worked in little smithies which are attached to, or part of their houses. Half inch or three quarter inch rod iron is used, and though sparrow bills are the main products, slate, clout and horseshoe nails are also made, and carried by the nailers by foot to cobblers and ironmongers in the Potteries.

The Home Office School farm became an Approved School in 1868. It was an old farm with two adjacent cottages – and a barn, which had been a chapel of ease in which the Vicar of Caveswall formerly held services. It was entirely the conception of Mr J E Davies, Stipendiary Magistrate for the Potteries. It was supported by Mr James Edwards, who contributed £200 towards the scheme.

It was opened in January 1870, with two boys and was managed very efficiently by Mr Benjamin Horth. It is still there in the 21st century and has gone through many name changes and different authorities governing it. It now holds 120 boys up to 15 years old. There they receive an elementary education with a strong practical bias – gardening, woodwork, metalwork and pottery plus some pre-vocational work in farming, gardening, domestic and maintenance work.

There's another chapel, a bit higher up, at the highest point of the main road. The chapel is known as Mount Zion. It was built in 1812. The main door is right opposite the Mile Stone Marker (that is still there). In this chapel the seats are actually rented and, in 1873 the rent varied from 9d to 3 shillings and 9d. Most people couldn't afford this rent. A Sunday school was built at the side of it in 1868.

I often try to remember what Werrington was like before I was transported back to the 19th century. It's hard to remember now as it's been so many years. However, standing at the highest point of the village is the Windmill – not the pub of the same name, but the windmill itself. It is said to date from 1730. Mark Greatbach was the last person running it as a mill. In the 21st century it's no longer in use and the wind veins have been dismantled, it being just a sorry sight of its former self. From what I heard, when moving to Werrington in 2016, it had been taken over by the local platoon of the Home Guard in 1940 who, after some gutting and re-construction, castellated it and used it as their headquarters.

Of course, ahead in the 21st century, a little community of stone houses, in Washerwall, still existed, but the well was dry. I don't know when it dried up but it couldn't have been too long before I came to Werrington as I'd seen previous notices of well dressings. These were fancy affairs with the children dressing up. A local dignitary would come and give a speech and the local vicar would be there to bless the water. There would be a fair with all sorts of goodies made and sold. Of course, when the well dried up, there would be no water to bless and that was the end of the Washerwall well-dressing.

The little row of cottages, where my cottage stood, was gone by the 21st century and been replaced by modern houses, built up a steep bank, actually on top of the quarry. They had been built with a multitude of steps leading up to the front doors. I remember counting that one of the houses had 33 steps at the front – a bit of a task for the postman and too bad if you wanted something large delivered or had a child in a pram! The person who designed them should have been shot.

In the 19th century, the parish of Werrington didn't actually exist, as such. Apart from the hamlet of Washerwall, there were just a few houses – a pair of cottages at the main road end of Washerwall and a few cottages by the windmill and Windmill pub, a bit further along in the direction of Cellarhead. The Post Office near the junction of Johnstone Avenue (now moved further down towards Bucknall and combined with a Bargain Booze shop), was a pub too, The Blue Boar, and there were a further four pubs on each corner of the Cellarhead junction – what's there now is a health centre and an Indian restaurant, The Mantra.

The Washerwall that I know now, in the 19th century, is just a dirt track, with two quarries in total. From my memories of the 21st century, the road is a properly tarmacked road with houses all along, and a parade of shops, including a Co-op. Turning into the main Cellarhead to Hanley Road (Ash Bank) you have a chemist, a library and a GP surgery. St. Philip's Church is over Ash Bank, next to which is the church hall, where numerous events take place, including table tennis, yoga, dancing, a painting class, etc. There is also a little parade of shops in Johnstone Avenue. All this to cater for the new parish of Werrington, which first began to be built around 1960, when gas, electricity, running water and drainage were planned. Before that, there were no facilities as such in Werrington, apart from the facilities that the Meigh family had implemented to Ash Hall, and the numerous surrounding properties and farms they owned.

Washerwall hamlet borders Wetley Moor. Even on a warm sunny day, Wetley Moor has a dramatic appearance. I'd often found myself deep in the middle of the moor among the cattle that were allowed to graze there, and had no conception where I was and which way to go to get back to civilization.

There were many wells and springs and the water from Wash Well flowed down to Bucknall, joined by brooks and runnels from Hulme and Eaves and Ubberley. Spring Well (another well) had always been known for its sweetness and purity. From the sixteenth century strings of packhorses, laden with salt from Cheshire, drank from the springs – Salters Lane, which runs south from the traffic lights at Werrington, got its name as it was on the route taken by these packhorses carrying salt.

From the nature of their work and their proximity to the wild, wind-swept moor, this gave the residents a name for lawlessness and a reputation for toughness. The mines which were sunk and failed, brought to the district a population not over nice as to the means it employed to supply its necessities. Robberies of the most daring character are not infrequent; and even murders are known. Many farmers on their way back from market are waylaid and relieved of their purses. It is also said that there is a regular gang who make their living by this kind of thing.

It's not only danger to travellers being robbed or killed on the Moor but the surface is riddled with old shafts and stone holes. I had been told the story of Rev E. Powys, a rector of Bucknall, who had been riding over the moor one day, when his horse stumbled and he was thrown over its head. When he regained his feet, he found that his horse was nowhere to be seen. It had fallen down a disused shaft sixty feet deep! Contemplating this, reminded me of what could have been back in 1842, when Job Meigh was chasing my John, on horseback, over the moors and Job whipped my John off his feet and into one of these shafts. Of course, that never happened as my future had divided back in 1842. If I'd chosen to stay in the 21st century, I would have found the bones of John down this shaft, but I decided on the path of another future, to stay with John, so John is with me now in 1881. There's no way I could have told John all of this, but he found out some of it anyway - and that's why he left me – he couldn't concede that I could possibly have come from the future - that was just too unbelievable, and his only reasoning for the stories he'd heard, was that I was insane and he, therefore, chose to leave me.

I went to check on John. He had gone back to sleep and, with the heat of the fire, I found myself falling asleep too.

CHAPTER 6 – BUCKNALL

I was dreaming of my rounds as a nurse and midwife. It was a fitful dream, jumping from one thing to another. Back in the day, the little children born were so small, they looked like little old men and women with hollow cheeks and big eyes. There was just not enough food to eat. Work was on and off and, if the man of the house got ill, all the family suffered. I would collect all the newspapers and clean rags to take on confinements. My dream calmed as I remembered that things are a little bit better now.

My dream flitted onto Old Mrs Green, the nurse I learnt so much from, had passed onto me her tips for using natural herbs for healing. Of course, some of these have been refined and made into tablet form or for intravenous injections, although natural remedies are still being used. We are still in Victorian times and medicine hasn't really advanced that much by 1881. Prince Albert did a lot for the country at the beginning of Victoria's reign. He wasn't allowed to deal in the politics of the country, so decided to take upon himself schemes to enrich the lives of the poor and attempts to build up trade - the Great Exhibition, being the climax of his endeavours. However, following the death of her beloved Albert, Victoria has hidden herself away from public view, only being seen fleetingly, completely encased in black, and the people are quite upset at her seeming unwillingness to meet her people.

I was half awake, dozing, thinking - still, life goes on in her absence and science is making great strides in all aspects of industry and medicine. We still haven't much in the way of cures, apart from the quack remedies. The great medical discoveries are just on the horizon, but not with us yet, and - I found, and still find, these herbal remedies quite effective.

My dream flitted from Queen Victoria wearing black, back to Mrs Green at her whisky-making still she used to make natural herbal oils. I was lucky enough to get this still before she died. It meant that I would have to scour the countryside and rocky areas where these plants grew. I got to know where to look for them and when.

I found myself awake, dozily thinking of the herbal cures Mrs Green had taught me. Motherwort is a good one. It is meant to be used for female troubles but can also help men. I use it to soothe anxiety in pregnant women and for post-natal depression – also to aid expelling the afterbirth. Mrs Green made it clear to me that it was not to be used until labour had actually commenced, but it could be used to ease early labour pains if they begin prematurely. She insisted it should not be taken with blood thinners, such as willow-bark (containing the main ingredient of Aspirin), or people with clotting disorders. So I couldn't give this to my John.

It can also alleviate the restlessness, anxiety, tension and insomnia some women experience during labour. Postnatally, it is given to help the uterus relax and return to normal.

Motherwort acts as a uterine tonic, which helps to regulate menstruation, bring on delayed periods and can reduce and smooth muscle cramping, particularly menstrual cramps, reducing premenstrual tension and discomfort. Most menstrual cramps are partially due to inadequate circulation in the pelvis. Motherwort may help calm menstrual pain by both reducing spasms in the uterus and improving blood flow to the pelvis.

To prepare Motherwort I cut and dry the herb and make a tea, using 1-2 teaspoons per cup of boiling water, and leave to infuse for 10 minutes. Three cups can be had per day. The tea can be sweetened with a little honey. The smoke from burning a little in the fire also helps to settle stress. The herb acts as an antispasmodic to relax muscles, including the heart. It slows heart palpitations and a rapid heartbeat, making it an excellent remedy for cardiac anxiety – decreasing blood pressure and improving heart circulation. I find it helpful also with people suffering grief, anger and general upset. It has so many curative qualities, even helping to decrease cholesterol and prevent blood clots forming.

Another good herb is Lovage – useful for toothache and sore gums.

It smells somewhat like celery when crushed. Its leaves are used as a herb, the roots as a vegetable and the seeds as a spice. I use it for patients suffering from inflammation, indigestion, joint pain and headaches and an anti-histamine – that, eventually, reduces the body's allergic response and helps alleviate itchy eyes, runny nose and other serious allergic reactions . The root is thick, fleshy, greyish brown and carrot-like. It produces pale yellow flowers in summer followed by small, yellow-brown and highly aromatic fruits. I find it helpful also for patients suffering from gout, arthritis, and haemorrhoids, and it helps soothe upset stomachs caused by poisons and other dangerous infections. I find that direct application of Lovage leaves, or as a salve, can assist with decreasing symptoms of psoriasis and acne, and promoting smoother and better-looking skin. Quite a few of my elderly female patients ask for this to improve the look of their wrinkles!

Apart from this, this amazing herb actually contains eucalyptol and I find it very useful for patients with respiratory problems – helping to loosen and expel phlegm. With so many patients working down the mines and dust inhalation in the potteries, this little herb is a marvel, as it can help reduce lung inflammation and irritation and promote rapid healing. It is most helpful for children with colic. Not only this but, because of its high nutrient density, it has a potential to improve kidney health and soothe severe side-effects of menstruation such as cramps and bloating when taken at the beginning of a menstrual cycle. It possesses carminative properties that may address bloating and excess gas by reducing bowel irritation and promoting healthy and normal movement in the colon. It can assist with relieving intermittent fevers and feverish attacks and helps get rid of body toxins through the skin.

I use it to aid coughs, abdominal pains and even heart problems, and as a herbal remedy for jaundice and liver complaints. It is a natural diuretic to relieve kidney stones, can be used as a blood cleanser and as a treatment for conditions like, skin eruptions, gout rheumatism, malaria, pleurisy, boils, migraines and aching throats.

You can eat the leaves in a salad and the stems can be candied as a sweet treat. I grind up the seeds, using a mortar and pestle and add as a spice or seasoning to breads and biscuits prior to baking. Using Mrs Green's still, I can make up an oil to be added to a bath, or massage oils. However, again, this is another herb that cannot be used on pregnant women or people taking anticoagulant medicines like Warfarin, plus patients are advised not to go out in the sun.

Elderflower and Coltsfoot has to be bruised and made into a tea. Coltsfoot is used for treatment of bronchitis, lung cancer, emphysema, inflammation, rheumatism, swelling and water retention, tuberculosis. and coughs. Again, a brilliant little herb to help with my coal-miner patients. I used the leaves and flowering buds. Again, these two herbs are not to be used for pregnant patients or those with liver disease and to be used cautiously with blood thinners or antiplatelet agents, e.g. willow bark (aspirin).

William Herliston was one of my patients. He'd been a coalminer all his life and, in 1861 was in his early 70s. He was a poor old guy, with nothing to show for a life of hard toil. He'd had to give up work now, though. The coal dust had finally got down to the last bit of his lungs and he could just about breathe, coughing and spluttering and hardly able to talk. Also, the weight was dropping off him and he was left little more than skin and bones. What a life, no pension, no payment from his firm for ill health, and expected to work until you drop. I would visit him as often as I could to make the Elderflower and Coltsfoot preparation for him and make him as comfortable as possible. It seemed to ease his cough, so he could get some sleep. I'd also make a warm salve of Lovage to put on his chest. Of course, he didn't last much longer and I provided him with morphine for his last struggling days. There probably wasn't much a doctor could do in the 21st century, except a lung transplant. It was strange that younger coalminers didn't seem to show the signs of lung damage until they got into late age but, even if they'd given up going down the pits, they would still develop the disease in later life. Of course, some were lucky and got away with it altogether. I suppose that would be down to the genes.

Of course, there are the normal colds and splutters over the winter months but sometimes these advanced into full-blown influenza, especially with the very young and elderly. I advise them to keep warm and wrap up well . For the little ones I make candied stems of Lovage, which they adore. Elderflower is for the treatment of influenza -. 2 or 3 teaspoons of syrup taken 4 times a day for 5 days- cooked. It has to be cooked, otherwise it can cause vomiting and diarrhoea with possible cyanide poisoning – so not something to be meddled with.

Then there are poppy seeds. Unripe seeds when scored, exude a milky latex – this is the morphine and codeine, and highly addictive, but are good for pain, even birth pains. I make the seeds into a paste to spread around the patient's gums, where it is absorbed. As it happens, chloroform is readily available to assist with the pain of childbirth, and I had a supply from Dr Knight.

Victorian women might be almost continually pregnant, between marriage and menopause. Childbirth is risky and painful. These God-fearing people of Staffordshire widely believe that labour pains are imposed by God because Eve had sinned in the Garden of Eden and that they should bear the pain, sometimes biting down on a piece of wood. There is no gas or air but, thankfully for Queen

Victoria agreeing to be administered chloroform during childbirth, it had, some time ago, become respectable to have this administered as an anaesthesia. Dr Snow had discovered chloroform. He was the same man who discovered the source of cholera in a London epidemic.

There is also Rupture Wart, brilliant for bad wounds and deep cuts. It only grows in sandy places and gravel. I can only go looking for it on a hot summer's day, as the flowering plant has to be dried quickly, in the shade. and it cannot be stored. The herb has a slightly bitter taste. I make this into a poultice to be pressed on the wound before stitching. It has an astringent element to it. I also use it in treatment of upper respiratory tract infections, arthritis, rheumatism and as a blood-cleansing agent as it has mild anticonvulsive and disinfectant effect on the urinary tract and prevents formation of kidney stones. You can make a tea of it, using one teaspoon of the herb to hot water and allowing it to steep.

I fell back into my dream. In 1870 there was a lady, Mrs March, who lived at 43 Roggin Row, Bucknall. She had had child after child and was pregnant again. These houses were the poorest in Bucknall. On a visit to her she pleaded with me, "Oh nurse – Ah'm wi' child agin. We're clemmed as eet is en thrutched ite, en ah'm so wanky. Ah conna 'ev anuther babbie. Whut am ah gonna do? Is there nowt yer con do to git reed of eet fer may? Ah mayne, ah've onnly just 'ad a babbie en his sen ayven browght in 'is brothers two childer en woif to live wi' us, 'en shay's not warking either, just living off us. Ah dunna blayem 'im, 'is brother dayed dine the moin en the woif's seek en conna manage."

I looked over at the poor mite – a little girl called Olive. She was lying in a drawer that had been removed from the chest of drawers and lined with a blanket. They couldn't afford a cot or cradle.

Mrs Jones continued, "Way dus oor best. En oor Mary, follows the local cowl curts traiying te knuck payces off te breng wom. The carter ne'er says nowt as shay'd gee 'im whut fer. May en George, well way tries te git a few coppers som 'o the tarm, busking itesayd factory geetes."

"Sorry, Mrs Jones, I understand the financial situation you are in but I'm not willing to do a termination, however, I will ask Dr Knight. It may well be against his ethics though."

"Beggin' mar longuidge, noss, but sud 'is ithics. Thus babbie'll kell us o. Eet's not fayre, anuther babbie yayre efter yayre en nay fooed en nay monney. Mar George dunna git much wark, eet's paycemail loik. Mar girl, Hannah brengs in a beet, shay's a potter – shay's 12 neow en mar sun, William – 'es a yong mon neow, 'es 17 en a kerter but both his sen en yong William, will theer dine pub, spinding whut lettle thee arns, afore ah've got ony. T'uther childer - thah's Mary - oo's 8, George - oo's 7, Alice - oo's 3 – will theer o at schooel, thun theer's lettle Sarah, oo's 2, Olive an' ol, oo's no yit a yayre owd. Es thah nowt yer con di? 'E just wunna layve may alowne. Ah've 'eerd theer's sommit colled Penny Royal thut'll sheft a babbie but ah've trayed eet whun ixpicting oor youngest en eet dinna wark. Ah wu worrit reet through in keese God puneshed may. Ah ixpicted sommit cod bay wrung wi' mar babbie. Lockily shay wus olraight."

"Yes, your little girl is fine, thank goodness, although a bit underweight."

Ah've 'eerd too theer's summit colled Slipper Elm, som wemmen uses thut. Thah uses a stayl knetting naydle."

"Please, please do not go down that road. You will harm yourself and get an infection. You could die. I've seen women who have done this and they've ended up in hospital and died. You don't want to leave your family without a mother, do you? No, don't even think about it. Has your husband not thought of using condoms? I know they're hard to get hold of, and basically under the counter, but I will ask Dr Knight if he can get hold of some for you. He may be able to get some on prescription or even send over to America for them. You will have to pay though and, of course, that's where the problem lies, you have no money. I do really feel sorry for you. Have you tried the withdrawal method, although it's by no means a great preventive method, or try to prevent your husband going anywhere near you except just before or after your monthly."

"Ah'll tray, but somtarms theer's nowt stupping 'im."

"Well, just ask him if he wants you to die and to be left with all of your children to care for. See what his answer is to that. Tell him Nurse Knight told you and to see me if he needs to ask any questions." and I left her to ponder this. I was using the name, Nurse Knight, after John left me. People had started calling me that after I started working with Dr Knight and I just didn't correct them.

I left her some lavender, which has a calming effect when burnt.

That memory woke me up - it was distressing. I looked over to John. he was still sleeping soundly. My mind was restless and I couldn't get into a good sleep pattern. My thoughts started to drift to the Bucknall area, where I did, and still do, a lot of my nursing.

Saturday nights are the worst in Bucknall and Hanley. It isn't a place to be, especially when they all turned out of the pubs and I try not to be out late, but babies don't choose when it is convenient to come into the world. The men will be out in the streets shouting and singing, after spending all their wages. This often develops into a scrap or two and you can hear the sound of the men's clogs as they, stagger up the road. All is then quiet for a bit then the damndest row, doors banging, women screaming, children crying, running out of the houses in their shifts and vests. Some of the men get so mad drunk that they turn their wives and children out into the streets. They have to sleep in the closet or at a neighbour's – anywhere they can find. Once I'd settled the new mother and new born, I'd wait until the coast was clear before making my way back home.

See, a pub is a place of rest and charity to customers. They have no coal fire at home, some of them would never have had a meal only for having a generous publican. So, the men sit in the pubs waiting and drinking, and never bother about food. Some landlords are good and supply cheese and bread for their customers. One of these pubs is the Cat in Keeling Lane, Northwood. The Northwood Arms hadn't been built yet, nor the housing around. The Northwood Arms is a pub I visited every so often in the 21st century and I understand from publications that Mr Sheratt owned the pub in the early 20th century and would take in kiddies overnight, who had been thrown out by their drunken fathers. The publicans would make a fuss of the men.

Most think nothing of their women back home, and whether they have food or not. Women work, washing, cleaning, patching, mending, anything to feed their children. Some women work in the "biscuit" on pots to get money. Some go to Hanley market and ask the butcher for something rough and cheap for the dog, then bring it home and cook it for the kids, it is either that or starve, they can't do anything else.

If they have no coal, they are not be able to light a fire, and so, are not able to cook. You have to light a fire to cook, as there is no gas. Instead, they eat sandwiches – bread and cheese, bread and dripping, jam, lard anything cold. I found myself dozing again and having a remembered conversation with a young boy, Arthur, out in the street in Keelings Lane. He was telling me that the local families would get "a 'pennoth' of chips between them all on bread a half-penny cake as a treat. "Afore schooel way weet fer cowl curts goin' te putbonks. Way knuck payces eff the bock to tack wom fer ma's fayre. Oor faithers'll go int' pub o deey whar eet's werm. Oos childers weet fer warkers goin' wom at neet en cadge ony fooed thah've no aten or way tray te get cuppers bay deein' ony irrands. Ah've tacken wushin' frum 'anley op Birches 'Ed Leene te Kerry 'Ill te a beeg firm ise. Way goss mailes tacckin irrands, tarm dunna kynt. Ma wod saye, 'Ah want yer wom arly, tack a beesin, go dine Grand 'Otel in 'Anley, say ef thah've got ony drepping. Three pennoth o' drepping is yommy. Eet oozes uff the mate the toffs 'an fer theer males – eet's gooed stoff. Yer say, ma canna afford bay a jynte te cooek te git drepping fram uf eet."

I was awake again. I couldn't help but feel sorry for these families. My thoughts wandered to Northwood. In 1850 the population of Northwood was 3,300 mostly made up of pottery workers. It stretched from Providence Square along Keelings Lane through Upper Green, skirting Birches Head along to Far Green – old names that have lost their meaning.

The district used to have its own constable, but the job became so dangerous that policemen had to patrol in pairs. One of the most popular constables is 'Bobby' Shenton. It is said that he can look after himself 'very well if you please'; but his popularity came from being able to look the other way when indiscrete behaviour might otherwise bring him into conflict with his neighbours.

One part of Northwood which has achieved notable infamy is West Street, which lies in an area below a few yards of derelict land called 'The Rocks' bordering on Eastbourne Road; in the 21st century, it is a familiar and pleasant boulevard alongside the public park. It is here that women of ill-repute gather on the Sabbath to ply their trades which is a magnet for the local Hanley lads and rough clients. These are 'shilling women' who charge even less when beer has fired them. There are enough public houses to sink the proverbial battleship –fifteen – almost one for each head of the household.

It is claimed by the constabulary that the Northwood women are far more deadly than the Northwood men in the course of regular street fights, usually over money, payment in kind, jealousy and spite.

The Cat Inn in Keelings Road is indeed an ancient inn. While the other 15 pubs in Northwood arrived as a result of beer-house legislation in 1830's the Cat Inn has been there long before that. In fact it is well attested that men would turn out for a round of cock fighting from the end of the 18th century until well into Victorian times.

I drifted into sleep, remembering a conversation I'd had with Arthur about the comings and goings at the Cat in the 1840's.

"You could probably buy anything in the Cat for the right price and no questions asked nor answers expected. There was a scruffy bloke who'd come round with a dirty sack and tip out seven or eight joints of beef on the bar. Filthy and black as coal they were. But my father would always buy one for a shilling to take home for the weekend. Mother would wash all the dirt off and come Sunday it tasted lovely roasted with all the trimmings. Of course in those days meat was very scarce. I remember sometimes my mother would stuff a butterfly's heart and carve it up with lettuce for sandwiches!" Obviously that was tongue in cheek, but gives an idea of the starvation rations people had to survive on.

My dream then turned to a little shop in Bucknall. I take advantage of visiting the shop, whenever I am there, mainly as it seems to sell everything – things I cannot get at the little shop in Washerwall. It is at the top of William Street – owned by Mr Pennington. . It is packed full. There are bundles of sticks and firelighters stacked behind doors, shelves full of bags containing, flour, sugar, oatmeal, candles, oats, matches, grate polish, Beechams pills, Epsom salts, (which I find useful for helping wounds to heal), tobacco, cigarettes, babies dummies and all other sorts of items.. On the wooden counter is normally placed a lump of streaky bacon, a slab of butter and a chunk of cheese, next to the scales. The shop wouldn't pass any hygiene laws. In the misty window unwrapped sweets, chocolates, liquorice sticks, monkey nuts with a big grey cat lying amongst it all. There was a paraffin tank. You take your own bottle for paraffin. Mrs Pennington draws it out of the tank with a sort of pump and her hand always shakes so half of it goes back in the tank. Her excuse is, as always, that her nerves are bad that day but really, it is to give you short measure. She then rub her hands, wet with paraffin, through her hair. This she claims keeps her hair healthy and stops her catching cold.

The first time I went in, I happened to notice, on one of the lower shelves, bottles of arsenic – readily available over the counter! "What are you keeping arsenic for" I asked Mr Pennington, trying to sound nonchalant and just interested, also trying to suppress my feeling of angst at the thought that anyone, even children, could so easily purchase such a dangerous drug.

He smiled as he replied, "Oh, begging yer pardon, but way 'as some ladies come in as want arsenic to remove, if yer dunna mayned may saying - superfluous 'air. Thee also comes in for rat poison and uses it to kill kitchen flies." As I'd raised my eyebrows, which he interpreted as a look of interest, he continued. "Jest for want of saying, dust thou know that all those floral wallpaypers yous ladies loik, well the grane colour is made of arsenic. Thut goes fer the grane fithers in the fancy 'ats theer fond o'. Eet's used wereld-wide. Ah've 'eerd seey thut way British 'an bin accoosed bay the Frenchies o' poisoning Napoleon, bay decorating 'is prison on St. 'Elena wi' grane-patterned wa'paper. Well ah nivver. Gooed reedance to 'im. Gooed jub don. Ah wodna bay sayn jed wi' grane wallpayper – or mebbie ah wod." And he laughed.

I couldn't help but think how easy it would have been for a desperate wife to murder her husband – there'd been a few tales of such murders, those plus the acid bath murderer. Another thought came to mind that the floral wallpapers in prosperous parlours, and the brilliant leaves on fashionable hats, could kill the workers who had close contact with the arsenic in the green dye and there was no retribution. In those days Victorian employers had no duty to safeguard the health of their employees.

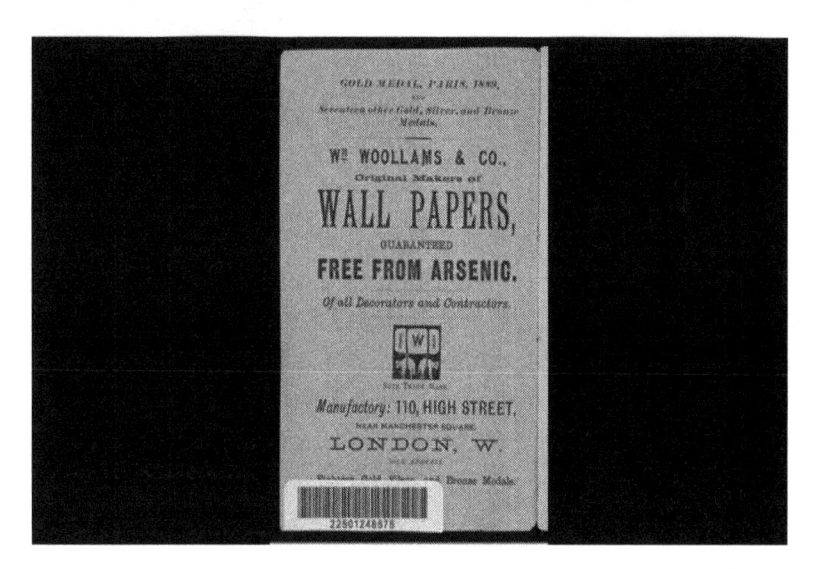

GOLD MEDAL, PARIS, 1889,

Seventeen other Gold, Silver, and Bronze Medals.

W<u>M</u> WOOLLAMS & CO.,
Original Makers of
WALL PAPERS,
GUARANTEED
FREE FROM ARSENIC.
Of all Decorators and Contractors.

Manufactory: 110, HIGH STREET,
NEAR MANCHESTER SQUARE.
LONDON, W.

On subsequent visits to this little shop I saw an advertisement for Crane's little bon-bon pills for sluggish liver and "a beautifier of

102

the Complexion". I dreaded to think what evils were contained in this concoction. On asking Mr Pennington if I could examine the bottle, he said he didn't stock them. There was just a private address on the advert – so a heavy hint that no chemist would actually stock them.

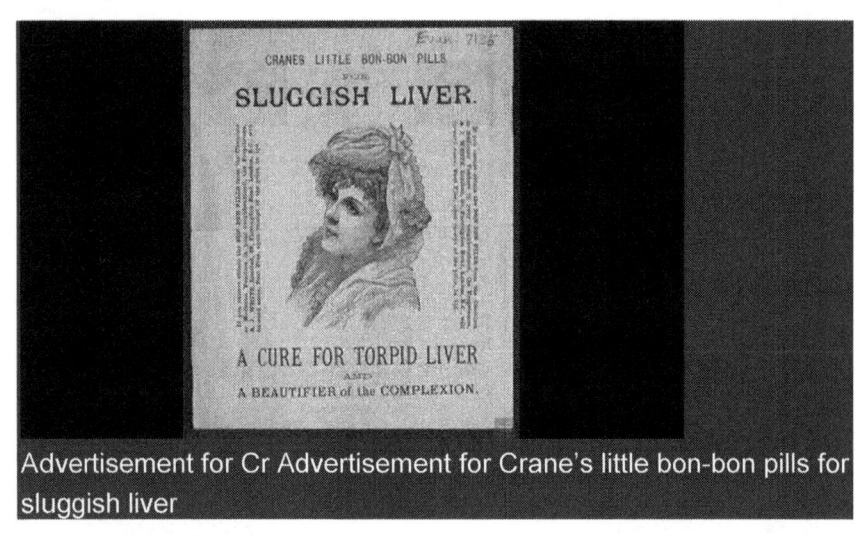

Advertisement for Cr Advertisement for Crane's little bon-bon pills for sluggish liver

Looking around the shop further, I also noticed a bottle of Dr James's Fever Powder. This I found out contained antimony and ammonia in toxic amounts. Anderson's Scots Pills for indigestion would cause piles and chronic constipation. Steel's Aromatic Lozenges promised to 'repair the evils brought on by debauchery' (a veiled reference to syphilis), but resulted only in a painful and dangerous inflammation.

Dr Collis Browne's Chlorodine was marketed as a remedy for indigestion, but came in useful for almost anything, unsurprisingly since it contained a hefty dose of morphia, as well as kaolin for stomach pains. I used that with patients as I remember having it myself when I was growing up and it did the trick, causing no ill-effects. Morrison's Pills resulted in numerous deaths – and a fortune for the maker. Several 'remedies' for babies' wind, such as Godfrey's Cordial, contained opium, which certainly quietened querulous infants, but overdoses could be fatal, especially when combined with gin.

Chloroform was useful in an attack of toothache. Or the sufferer could try morphia, or laudanum, another derivative of opium. They could all be bought from chemists, no questions asked.

I was naturally very wary as to what was contained in any of these preparations before using any in my nursing rounds. I would use only natural preparations if I could, such as olive oil for earache, a teaspoonful of warm olive oil poured onto cotton wool and plugged into the affected ear.

I was asked once to look at a little boy, Jeremiah Beardmore. He was only five, but had earache and applied this warm olive oil solution to his ear. The infection soon cleared up and he was back giving his mother a merry dance.

Another story came into my dream. It was early 1857. I was going out to visit a woman at Kerry Hill. She lived on a little farm there. She'd got four children and was due to give birth to another.

I knocked on the door. "Hello, Mrs Brown, it's the midwife, Nurse Knight, coming to see how you are." There was no answer so I started to look around the farm buildings. I found her clattering around in the cow house. She looked in a distressed state and I could see that she must have had the baby.

"Oh, so I've arrived too late. You've already given birth. You should be resting, not working here. Here, sit down. How did the delivery go? I would like to check the new baby, make sure it's alright and thriving, Mrs Brown. Is it a boy or a girl?"

Mrs Brown carried on working, ignoring me.

"Come on, Mrs Brown. I need to inspect the baby. I waited a bit, but still with no response. Look, Mrs Brown. If you don't answer me I will have to report it…… that's when I noticed that Mrs Brown was crying.

"There, there, hush, Mrs Brown. Sit down" and she carried on weeping onto my shoulder as I knelt beside her.

"Obviously, something has gone wrong and you have had a terrible shock. But, please, you need to tell me where the baby is."

"Eet wus born jed, eet wodna braythe. Ah 'ad te 'ide eet frum t'other childers, I dinna want 'em sayin' body en gittin' opset. Sa ah 'id eet. Eet's o'er thah." She was pointing in the direction of the well, so I got up and walked, tentatively, towards the well. Mrs Brown followed slowly behind me. I didn't know what I would find, although I'd seen enough bad things in my time but still felt my heart beating a little faster.

"Dine theer, int' well." she indicated.

I looked down and saw the body of the baby, surrounded by straw, in the bucket. I immediately started hauling the bucket up and grabbed hold of the baby. I gave it a wipe over with the straw to clean it off and that's when I noticed that the boy was breathing.

"Mrs Brown, the baby's alive. You have a wonderful baby boy." I shouted, with relief. The straw must have kept it warm. Mrs Brown cried tears of joy then and went to fetch a blanket to wrap the boy in. I was so relieved and happy for her. She named the boy Joseph.

My dream then turned to a family I'd known, who lived at 149 New Bucknall Road in 1851, the Bennett's. They weren't a large family, four daughters and one son. The two older daughters were painters in a pottery and the son was a potter.

I'd been called to the family as both daughters, Caroline (aged 17) and Sarah (aged 15) were showing signs of toxin poisoning. They worked in the "biscuit" on pots. Their fingers were wrapped in bits of rags and bleeding. The pots were rough without a glaze and they just wore all the skin away.

Caroline was worse. She was showing signs of lead poisoning, from the glazes used. She was irritable and said she felt tired all the time and had a cough. I was talking to her, asking about her work, but she seemed to lose concentration and couldn't follow what I was saying. I tested her hearing with the aid of a little bell from various distances and it appeared that her hearing was affected too. I asked her to hold her hands out straight in front of her, and there was a noticeable shaking of her hands. On questioning further it appeared she had also been suffering from diarrhoea and she was very slow in adding two numbers together or to remember what she had done the previous day. So, this was a sign that she was developing learning disabilities. I couldn't give a blood test as I would have wanted to – blood tests had not been invented. The development of medicine at the time was basic, and often contrary to the health of the patient – they were still using leaches to 'bleed' a person. We were basically, at this time, still in the middle ages.

I knew that toxins could be ingested, inhaled or absorbed through skin cuts. I advised both of the girls, firstly to leave that particular pottery. I knew Job Meigh had worked on glazes to remove the lead from them and had won a medal for services to industry – that was back in 1822. However, the new glaze hadn't been successful and he had continued working to improve his lead-free glaze.

I also advised the girls they had to make sure they followed my advice:

They were not to work again until their cuts had healed; not to eat at their tables; not to put any tools in their mouths; not to chew their fingernails; to put a cloth over their noses and mouths to protect them from the dust (there were no such things as respirator's or dust masks); to wash their hands thoroughly and to wipe their tables with a wet cloth instead of sweeping up the clay dust, at the end of every session.

Footsteps in the Past – The Secret

I got talking to the boy, John, just 12 years old, as I was bandaging his sisters' hands with a herbal poultice underneath made of chickweed. This was good for healing skin ailments.

The boy had been a potter since he left school, starting as a saggermakers bottom-knocker.

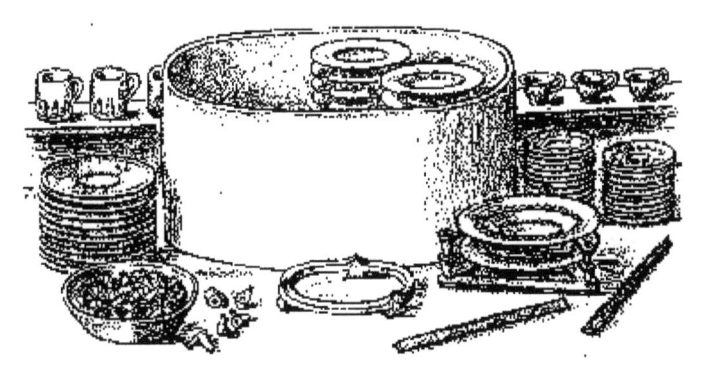

I found out from him that a saggar is a fireclay container, usually oval or round, used to protect pottery from marking by flames and smoke during firing in a bottle oven.

The saggar-maker, is a skilled man, producing the finished saggar, using his thumb to make a near join between the side and the base. The BOTTOM KNOCKER (a young boy) made the base of the saggar from a lump of fireclay which he knocked into Metal a metal ring using a wooden mallet or mawl (pronounced mow).

"Mar ma coms wi' may en seeys mar cousin wunted a lod, a saggermeekers buttom-knucker. Ah wint fer di thet. May fust jub wus te cut the clee and stack eet fer 'im. Way'd gorra concrayte bench en ah used te cut the clee wi' a sort of 'ay noif, cut eet in lengths fer the saydes o' the saggars. Ah'd knuck the clee solid with a mow in the iron freme. Eet wus bloomin' 'ard wark en yer far git a swit on. Ah then went onte tale slabbin' fer fayre greetes. Thay'se 'r painted bay the lasses but thus was onnly summer wark. Nayone wunts a taled greete in winter. So ah go te Johnsons pot bonk te find sommat else. Ah'v bin loadin' en unloadin' saggars, carryin' saggars on may yed wi' a roll. Yer put a roll betwixt the sagger en yer yed to tack the weight. Way med 'em frum women's stockings wrapped riyd en riyd taiight loik. Eet took prisure aff yer yed."

I was awake now, but didn't feel really refreshed because of my broken sleep. The sun was rising, so decided to get up. I'd get the washing done while John was still asleep. It looked like it would be a sunny day, although a bit windy, but that would help the washing dry. I would need to get the oven lit first to get hot water. It was a right chore, emptying the hot water into the wash barrel and heavy work turning the clothes and sheets around in the barrel, but it had to be done.

While occupied with the washing, and thinking back to my dreams, it occurred to me that I once did a survey of Keelings Lane. This was in 1851. It was just to see how many people worked in different trades in each family, including the children. The mothers normally were home-makers. What I found was that 70 people worked in the pottery industry, 1 was a grocer, one a joiner, 4 coal miners, 1 publican and 2 dress-makers. That's just one street, so a microcosm of the neighbourhood, showing the vast numbers working in the pottery industry.

As for the local coal mines, Hulme was classed as a hard mine. You couldn't make a living as the coal was too hard to get out. Next quality went to the pot banks for firing ovens and for household.

Coal off the Common was steam coal, Makin's pot bank had some.

The best coal was found at Bucknall. There was a pit up Dividy Lane by the Trent Tavern. Also one at Ubberley where they had to have a pump to draw the water off. It was keeping Hanley and Bucknall pits dry as well.

Northwood pit was a hot pit. You had to go down a big depth. It was sloping. They couldn't walk down as it was so steep. There they'd get a piece of leather and a piece of string, make a hole in the leather, put it under their behind, tie round the waist, one foot on the rail and the leather and they used to slide down. Then they had to pull them back up in a wagon. It was so hot and sweaty that the miner's shoes would rot and their feet were thick with blisters.

CHAPTER 7 – THE VISIT

It was the next morning. John was awake so I started preparing some breakfast for him. I had eggs and bacon but thought better of this, "not good for someone who's had a heart attack" I said to myself, so made some porridge with a dollop of honey on top. That would do and maybe a ploughman's lunch with sliced apple and possible a shepherd's pie with extra vegetables for tea. He hadn't eaten much for days and needed feeding up. It would last a few days and I would just have a taster with some veg and gravy.

John was feeling a lot better and could sit up without too much pain, and get to the rocking chair, but he was still very weak and couldn't stand for long.

I started talking to him about our time together, recalling the good times we'd had.

"Do you remember our wedding, John? We finally got married on 17th March of 1843. Mrs Meigh was kind enough to lend me one of her dresses, it was white with lace frills – quite lovely. Job Meigh and his wife were there, and a few of your work colleagues and, of course, Dinah, the cook at Ash Hall. I'd made a head garland of spring flowers."

"Yer, mar leedy, yer looeked booetiful."

"There was a bit of a to-do with Job Meigh though. He was asking where my parents were. I had to tell him my mother was ill and my father didn't want to leave her."

"Did yer mack thut oop? Ah've nivver sayn yer parents. They nivver cam te visit us. Ur thee stell aloive?."

"No, John, unfortunately, they have both died."

"Yer nivver telt may."

"No, and after a time, Job Meigh asked me again about them. I had to tell him they'd both died of the same sickness my mother had, cholera. I told him it was rife in London at the time."

"But yer dinna go te ony funeral. Woy deed yer seey nowt?"

"Well, I was pregnant by then, with our Alfred, and had morning sickness so I didn't really feel up to travelling. I didn't really want to go anyway, as we'd never been close."

"But whut abite 'is 'ise en belungings? Whut 'appened te thim?"

I had to think quickly, although I'd prepared beforehand, so long time ago, what I would say if this conversation ever came up. Reality was that my parents had died in 20th and 21st centuries respectively, before I'd ever come to Werrington.

"Well, to tell you the truth, I'd never contacted them about our wedding, so they didn't know anything about it. We'd been distant for so long, I just wanted to put them in the past and look to our future. They didn't even know where I lived. We'd had a big falling out and my father wanted nothing more to do with me. So, I suppose his estate was split amongst my parents' family – there were aunts and uncles and cousins. The money would have come in handy but, well….that was a long time ago now."

"Ah di rimember traying te ask yer, neow, but yer cheenged the sobjict - yer was sacretive en clommed up, so ah saed nay mer."

"That's right, so now you know. Anyway, we had our beautiful Alfred at the end of the year. We taught him everything we knew but he just wasn't academically-minded and preferred to be with his pals. No matter what I said, he insisted on doing mining. And look where we are now, wondering whether or not he's dead under the ground. Yes, I know you did everything you could to save him, almost killing yourself in the process, but it's the life he chose. Still, he married and has two lovely children. I'm hoping to hear from them. I've sent a message." I hung my head and a tear started to form…

John put his hand out to stroke my head. "Whut well bay will bay, Jane."

I recovered and continued. "He was such a precarious little chap, always getting himself into scrapes – a typical boy, and so interested in your building work. He wanted to follow you to work and climb your ladder. You let him try his hand at hammering a nail, remember?"

"Yer, thun 'e 'ommered 'is thomb, oh 'e deed yall, but 'e nivver geev op traying."

Just at that moment there was a knock at the door. "Who could that be" I said out loud, then "Come in, the door's open".

"Hello, ma." came the reply as Alfred's wife, Kate stood there with little Mary Annie and baby William in her arms."

I got up to give her a hug and help her with the baby. "Come, sit down. You've come a long way, all up that steep hill and carrying baby William too. You must be exhausted. Come, sit down and I'll make you a cup of tea."

John held his arms out to give her a hug. He sat up in the bed and Kate sat in the rocking chair with the baby. Little Mary Annie sat at the table and I gave her a juice and a pencil and paper to draw on.

I sat down beside John. John and Kate had obviously been talking while I made the tea but she turned to me as I entered the room. "He's gone ma." I got up quickly to give her a hug. "It's alright - I'm all cried out. I can't cry no more. It's been too long now and they can't get to everyone left down there. I've been over there. Roofs caved in after the explosion. It's a grave for our dear Alfred – 'is final resting place."

"Way feayred the woss, love, not 'avin' 'eerd onythen'." John added.

114

"Yes, I know 'ow much you tried to save 'im, dad, almost killing yourself by doing so. It was very brave of you, and foolish too, but I know you 'ad to try, and I thank you for trying. Luckily ma was able to save you and I'm not weeping over two people. There's gonna be a service of some kind at Bucknall Church this Sunday, if you're fit enough to go, dad."

"Ah'll git theer, bay sure o' thut. Som weey or tuther. Donna fret."

"Is there anything we can do to help you? I mean, you've got the two kiddies. What about food, money? How will you be able to manage? We'll help in what little way we can, naturally. Just say the word." I added.

"Oh, we'll get by, somehow or tuther. My ma lives in Bucknall. She said she'd be able to look after the children and, I suppose I'll have to get myself a job of some kind, maybe on the pots. I did a bit before I married Alfred and they're always crying out for more people. It won't be enough, as women aren't paid as much as the men for doing the same work. It's not fair, but that's how it is. It will be a struggle to pay the rent."

I felt really sorry for her. There really wasn't anything I could do. I was living from hand to mouth myself and had to be out all hours, sometimes, looking after folk. I'd given that all up for the time being to look after John, so there was no money coming in at the moment and, when I was back at work, Kate wouldn't really be able to depend on me to be available to help with the children, so I was really grateful that Kate's mother was available. There would be no compensation from the mine. If there was a disaster like this, or if you got ill, that was just too bad. There was no old-age pension – you worked till you dropped, and given the toxins found in the mines and potteries, that wouldn't be long – the average age of death for those working in the mines was 45. You had to be really fortunate, if that's the correct word, to still be alive in your 70s, after a life down the pit. In fact, if you'd got to your 70s, you'd still have to keep on working down the pit – as, as I said, there was no old-age pension. There used to be a poor fund in such circumstances, but the Government got rid of that in favour of the workhouses. They reckoned too many people were just working when they wanted and would rely on the poor fund when they didn't feel like working. The workhouse was now the only other option for people in dire straits. Families would be split apart into male and female sections and, if you were ill, you'd probably never get out again, apart from in a coffin. They'd put you in a uniform, like in prison. In fact the Chell workhouse had been nicknamed, "The Bastille". The work was hard, back-breaking work of breaking stones, or picking oakum out of old ropes. There were numerous rules and regulations, which were disobeyed at the inmate's peril. The food is nothing but poisonous-tasting gruel. You'd literally have to be at death's door to subject your family to the abject cruelty that went on these places.

Anyway, Kate and family finally went on their way and we'd agreed to meet them next Sunday at Bucknall Church. I added, "Please get a message to us if you hear any more or if you need anything urgently. I'll try to pop in to see you when I'm in the area, and see my little grandchildren." I smiled at Marie Annie and smoothed little baby William's hair, giving both of them a kiss.

"I will mum, pop, thank you." Kate said as we waved her off. She'd cope, with a little help from her friends and family. She was strong, but I could imagine the days of weeping she'd been through for her Alfred – I'd cried enough myself. They'd be no grave for her to mourn over, no gravestone with his name and dates on. The same applied to John and me.

CHAPTER 8 – GEOFFREY

Speaking to Kate about Alfred, and his almost certain death, just turned my mind to the other great loss in our lives. I didn't want to mention him - I was frightened to. It was too mind-blowing and would just disturb a nest of worms, especially with John in his weakened state, something that was just too sad to resurrect – something I did not want to speak about – something I was so ashamed of - the reason John and I had split up. John obviously saw how grave and ashen I'd become and must have realised that my thoughts had turned to our other son, something never far from his mind either. It was a subject that neither of us wanted to speak about - the proverbial 'elephant in the room'.

I heard John then softly say, "Geoffrey".

There, it had been said. His name had been spoken. I wanted to run away, to escape the torment of a trial that I assumed John obviously wanted to assault me with, just by saying his name. So many years I'd lived with the dishonour, the abject misery. Tearfully, I stuttered out, "He... he was such a lovely boy – so.... so completely different. He was a studious type.... took in everything that I said."

I continued, "I know how deeply hurt you were.... and still are- but it wasn't just you who suffered – I suffered ..... am still suffering."

"Jane, way nivver rayly tocked efter ah funt ite whut 'appened. Ah think way nade te go o'er ivverythin' agin, afore way con move on. A sort o' catharsis."

"But, it will only bring matters to a head again. I can see no use in going over old ground and coming to the same conclusion. I couldn't get through to you then, and I doubt I'll get through to you now. You've got your head in the sand. You'll only believe what you can prove, and you'll just get angry with me."

"Ah wunt te 'ear eet o agin. Ah nayd te." There was a touch of anger in his voice already. Obviously, he was feeling better, well enough for an argument that is, forgetting that he'd almost died and I had saved him. My attempts to bring friendship, or even love, back into our lives over the last few days, looked to have fallen on stony ground.

"Oh, John, it's so long ago, but still like yesterday in my heart. A hurt that's so deep. However, If you must. Don't be angry with me, please. It's been so many years and I've tortured myself every single day since." At this, it looked like John was about to get up and go, and I really felt that that would be him out of my life, yet again.

… OK." I took a deep breath…. "Remember, John, there were a few children from families around, who had money, so I had suggested to Mrs Meigh that I could possibly set myself up as a teacher. Mrs Meigh was very interested and helped me set up a little school in the nursery at Ash Hall. That was 1849."

Mrs Meigh was 64 at the time and, although she said she was still doing her exercises, following her stroke in 1842, she was finding things a little bit more difficult to get around, so I tended to think that she was not keeping to her routine so much. There was nothing I could do to force her to do the exercises, so let it ride. From what I gathered, there was still no improvement in her feelings towards her husband. He had caused her accident and there was no forgiveness there, and I didn't blame her. Job Meigh could be a right tyrant when he was in a mood and not to be affronted. I still remember him attacking me when I had offered to take minutes at one of his magistrate meetings just before the riots, as his brother, Charles, who normally took the minutes, was injured by pre-rioters, who'd gone to a coal mine to try to wreck it. I had taken the minutes in Pitman's shorthand. Looking at what he discerned as just scribbles, and not knowing that Pitman had set up shorthand courses (although, in fact, I had learnt my shorthand at school in the 20th century), he thought I was making a fool of him, and this after he'd gone out of his way to recommend my taking the minutes. He hit me violently, throwing me off my chair. He was pulled off me and it was explained to him about Pitman's courses. He was apologetic afterwards, but not until we were in the coach on the way back, but then he tried to make advances to me, which added insult to injury. and I threatened to leave his employment. He relented and asked me to stay on. So, that was Job Meigh, a brilliant man in all other respects and a philanthropist, but a violent man and seducer when roused.

"Anyway, John, I set up the school and even though the ages of the children ranged a fair bit, I coped, setting separate tasks in maths for each of the children, to match their age ranges. It was a good little school. I eventually taught English, with a smattering of French and German as well as history, geography and biology. The younger ones got a story while the older ones were doing maths exercises or something more exacting. Rote exercises were perfect for the kiddies learning their times tables, leading onto set exercises. This curriculum was somewhat advanced from what children normally learnt and I found, at first, that writing was the main task to be set. If any of them had attended a school before, it was a Sunday school where they were taught to read the Bible, but not in fact taught to write - they knew all the Bible stories but couldn't write them down.

These children, however, were the privileged few. As you know, children in the Potteries were taught from the age of 3 to 6 and, by 7 years old, they had to be out working in the Potteries. All they learnt at their pre-working schools were reading and a bit of arithmetic. They had no idea what was happening in the world, or history, or geography. It was thought such education was not needed and children should remain ignorant, just learn enough to get by in their jobs and their apprenticeships would teach them what they needed to do their jobs. That was it.

I continued, "Alfred and Geoffrey attended. Alfred was 6 and Geoffrey 5, then there was Gertrude, who was 8 in 1849 - she's the daughter of Job Meigh's brother, Charles. Little William Mellor Meigh, grandson of Job and Elizabeth Meigh was there. He was 7 – he's the son of William Mellor Meigh, the first, who's the son of Job Meigh and Elizabeth. His siblings came along too, Elizabeth, 10 and Annie, who was 5 at the time. His other siblings either hadn't been born in 1849 or were babies. Catherine was just 1 year old at the time, Ellen was born in 1850, Maria in 1852 and Marie Ann in 1856. There were also Anna, 6, James 8 and Thomas 10- children of Thomas Forester as publican in Bucknall and Jeremiah, 5, Ellen and Martha (twins – 7 years old) and Elizabeth, 8 – children of Jeremiah Beardmore, who was a farmer with 94 acres. Plus there was Thomas Cooper, 9, son of a Bucknall farmer with 150 acres."

I could see John listening intently, but he was getting a bit fidgety. He was obviously in some pain again, which was making him angry and moody. "Com on ducky, git on wi' eet."

I didn't like him calling my 'ducky'. I know it originated from the word 'duchess', but it wasn't 'love' or even 'mar leedy', as he had been wont to say. It was something you'd say to someone you didn't really know.

"Please bear with me John, I need to give you the setting. Anyway, I carried on with that for a few years. I suppose one day I was overly-tired, looking after the school, planning lessons, looking after the cottage and still dealing with any urgent nursing calls for my assistance, plus I think I must have been pregnant with Geraldine, although I didn't know at the time, so I wasn't thinking straight and was also feeling a bit nauseous. We were doing a history lesson, about Victoria and I happened to say that Victoria had gone into deep mourning following the death of Albert.

Most of the children didn't seem to pick up on this error – I don't know, they were probably not all that interested in history and were just day-dreaming, but our Geoffrey picked up his ears. I saw him start to put his hand up to say something, but then lowered it. He said nothing.

The next lesson was geography. We were talking about Germany, following on from Prince Albert having coming from Saxe Coburg. I was talking about the amalgamation of the individual German-speaking states into one Germany, some of which were Prussia, Bavaria, Saxony, Schleswig and Holstein, and the Frankfurt National Assembly of 1848. This was on-going at the time, so information was readily available in the papers. A proposed constitution was adopted for Germany on March 28, 1849. Germany was to have a unified monetary and customs system but each state would be responsible for its own internal affairs. Austria wasn't having any of this and wanted the entire Austrian Empire to enter or none at all. Frederick William of Prussia was elected new emperor of the Austrian Empire, but he refused the crown as he was too conservative to receive an imperial German crown from any hands except those of the other German princes. Prussia also rejected the proposed constitution. – I could see the younger kiddles' eyes closing at this and they were getting restless, and so was I, and just closed the lesson by saying something glibly, so unification of Germany isn't going to happen until Otto von Bismarck deliberately provokes the French into the French/Prussian war of 1870...... That's when Thomas Forrester put his hand up and asked me how I knew this. I flustered over the answer, finally getting out that that was just something that was bound to happen in the future, what with all the German/French aggravation, and that Germany would have to unite sometime in the future."

"So, 'ow ded yer knah thut?" John piped up angrily.

"You know, John. You just won't take it on board."

"Sa, thee o thowt yer a wetch tooe?"

"I'd prefer to say someone who can see into the future, John. There are people who can – take Nostradamus, who predicted centuries in advance, even the 2nd world war, calling Hitler 'Hissler.'"

"Yer et eet agin. Second werald wur? Yer barmy, a blitherin' eediot. Way've not 'ad ony 1st werald wur let alowyn ony 2nd wereld wur. Thut's why ah left ye. Blatherin' en fiellin' the kiddies yeds wi' eet."

"I'm sorry, I was tired. I made a mistake."

"Yer, med sich a midge-madge thut eet 'ad gotten oor Geoffrey killt. Eet was all along of you. Yer the raison 'es jed."

John made to get up to leave but didn't get far and fell to his knees. I went to help him up.

"Yer mithering may. Bogger uff. Efin ah cod ger ite o' 'ere, ah wod." I managed to help him back to the bed notwithstanding his attempts to try to shake me off.

I continued, "Yes, I'm the reason he's dead. Remember, it was you who wanted to go over all of this again John! Yes, Geoffrey had picked up on my second mistake too, but kept it to himself. He knew my secret. I'd told him. I made it out to be a fairy story of sorts - that his mother was a wizard come from the future just to have him and I could do all sorts of wizardry tricks and knew things that were going to happen, but I told him not to tell anyone, otherwise I might vanish back to the future. He laughed at the time but he never forgot it."

"Sa, ide 'e git kilt?" John said, grumpily, with his head lowered, breathing heavily. I could see how angry he was, but was trying to control his temper. I had some Aspirin already prepared, which I offered to him with in tea. My hands were shaking. He snatched it from me.

I made an effort to continue. "Geoffrey didn't appear that evening after school. He hadn't waited for me and gone off alone. I thought he was just going out to play and he'd come back when his tea was ready. But, by 6pm there was no sign of him and it was starting to get dark. You were back home by then and we both went out to look for him, calling his name over and over in the hopes that he would scurry out from behind a bush or wall, saying that he'd been playing hide and seek. It was dark now and we'd knocked on all of the neighbours' doors to ask if they'd seen him. No-one had, but seeing our distress, a few of them started searching with us, going off in different directions, with burning torches for lights. No-one knows how it happened, his poor bloodied body was found at the back of Ash Hall the next morning. Maybe he got in a fight, maybe with Thomas Forrester. Thomas was a lot bigger than him. I don't know..... Maybe Thomas was calling him names, saying that his mother was a witch and threw a large stone at him. These are all surmises because Thomas never owned up or said anything. I know he was very quiet for some time after – definitely not his usual self, but then he could have been grieving, for a school friend. Oh, John, yes, I own up – it must have been my fault that our poor little boy got killed."

John just grunted.

I was hanging my head in shame and wringing my hands, but got cold comfort from John. Anyway, I continued, sullenly. "There was a sort of inquest afterwards. Job Meigh, as magistrate, wanted to know the ins and outs of the case. The school children were questioned too and it eventually came out, after a lot of pressure from Job Meigh, what I had said about Bismarck and Prince Alfred."

Another grunt from John.

I continued, "Then Job Meigh interviewed me. He was at his worst, ranting and raving. He said, "I always thought there was something strange about you and now I know what it is. You're a habitual liar and deranged. Don't think I haven't had you checked out, you and your stories about your father having been a solicitor in Greys Inn Court in London. I thought it strange they didn't attend your wedding but, again, you made up a story, saying your mother was sick. Then, later on, you said they had both died. Oh yes, my girl, your chickens have come home to roost. Just to make you aware, missy - I had the necessity some little while ago of having to go down to London about a case being held there, and I took the opportunity of enquiring about a Mr Paget, who used to have offices in Greys Inn Court. I spoke with a few eminent, elderly

Footsteps in the Past – The Secret

gentlemen, who had been there for years and all shook their heads, denying they had ever heard of a Mr Paget. Now don't you go making up any other stories, saying that I've got the facts wrong – I DO NOT GET FACTS WRONG." He was shouting at me now. I was backing away, I thought he was going to strike out at me, as he'd done before, his hand was raised in the air. "Yes, get out of my sight. I've had enough of you, you good for nothing hag ……. I should have you arrested but I can't arrest you for lying. You've brought the death of your boy on yourself and you'll have to live with it – I think that's enough punishment for your lies. Go on, get out of my sight and off my land. You're not fit to be a teacher !.... - And I've never been allowed back into Ash Hall."

I was shaking now, remembering this incident.

John had turned his head away. He couldn't look at me. "Yer, Job Meigh telt it may hissen. 'E wunted to gee may the bag tooe, sa ah 'ad te git the story ite o 'im. Ah wus so flummoxed. 'E seyd 'ed onnly tack may beck effin ah laeft yer, en 'ad nowt mer te day wi' yer.... Ah mooched arint a beet, 'ad te think eet o'er, git may yed in order.... Eet wuz th'ardest chice ah ivver 'ad to mack. But, whut yer deed, thut wus tooe moch a beer. Sa, ah wint beck en telt 'im way wus feneshed."

"At least you left me the cottage, although I had to find a means to pay the rent myself. Yes, people needed a nurse but there was not much money to pay me. They would pay in kind, with milk and butter and bread, sometimes coal. They were hard times, but I got by. Of course, what made matters worse was that I found out I was indeed expecting our Rosalind. When she was born, I would

127

have to take the poor mite with me on my rounds, carrying her as well as my nursing equipment. You didn't want anything to do with her, so I registered her in my maiden name – Rosalind Paget. I taught her everything I know and she's grown up to be a remarkable young lady."

"Yer, ah've sin 'er arind." John said. His voice was just above a whisper with a notable rasp to it so I had to get closer to hear him.

"You won't have seen her recently, John. She went to London some years ago to train as a midwife. She's been at the London Hospital and is highly thought of. She's written to me and is attempting to set up a midwives' institute with three other nurses."

"Ah'm playsed shay's gittin' on." John said quietly, still with his head bowed down.

CHAPTER 9 - COMING OF THE RAILWAY

I wanted to cheer John up a bit, to get him out of this doldrum about Geoffrey.

"We had some good times, when we were together, John, didn't we? John lifted his head and gave a half smile. Obviously the Aspirin was working, and he was beginning to feel a bit better.

"Do you remember when the Bucknall Station was built? There was 'railway mania' around 1845 with track being built all over. Stafford, Crewe, Derby and Macclesfield were all connected. Everyone was so excited. They'd never seen anything like it and it meant that we weren't so cut off. Goods and pottery and clay and all sorts could be moved all over the country, imports and exports to and from the ports to and from other countries. Things were really looking up. There was an excitement in the air. Before, there was only the Trent and Mersey Canal, which took ages to move anything by barge. Of course, the Trent and Mersey Canal had a railway line from 1776, but this was something else, far greater."

John interrupted, "Yer, ah wus eenterested in thus tooe. Theer war two companies thut promoted routes – The Churnet Valley Reelweey gittin' a lane frum Macclesfield to Derby wi' a branch te Stoke en the Staffordshire Potteries Reelweey wi' a route frum Macclesfield te the Grand Junction Reelweey meenlane at Norton Bridge wi' a spur te Crewe."

"But the Potteries still didn't have a railway."

"Frum what ah rimember, thays two companies jined furces en Parliament approeved a scame to amalgameet wi' the Trent Valley Reelweey, which beckem the North Staffordshire Reelweey. Payple started colling eet The Knotty. Thah then built The Pottery Lane, te run frum a junction wi' the Manchester en Birmingham reelweey at Congleton te the Grand Junction Railway at Colwich, te breng the reelweey Tunster, Bursley, 'Castle, 'anley, Stock, Fenton, Longton en Stonn. The Churnet lane wus built te run frum Macclesfield through Leek, Cheadle en Toxeter te jine the Midland Reelweey lane betwane Burton-upon-Trent en Derby sa way gorra direct link 'twane Manchester en Derby."

"Yes, do you remember, we went to the official 'cutting of the first sod' ceremony? It was in a field in Etruria. It had been really dry – September 1846 I believe. We left little Alfred with a neighbour as we didn't know what to expect. As it was, the field was packed with people and all sorts of dignitaries."

"Yer, ah rimember. Thah'd 'ad a ropped aff area fer directors en lowds of uther invaited guists."

"Yes, but before getting into the field, we had followed a procession, along with a huge crowd of people. John Lewis Ricardo, the Member of Parliament for Stoke and Chairman of the 'Knotty' was at the head of the procession, taking about a mile-long route through town."

It was good to see changes that had been made to the area as I didn't get a chance to go to Hanley much. There was gas lighting for a start, although few and far between, and there wouldn't be gas lighting in homes until 1865, and then only about half of the houses had gas."

Yes, I thought to myself, sewage was still a problem at the time. Shelton Highway Board had built some early in the 1850s but it was some years before the problem of sewage disposal was tackled. In the meantime Fowlea Brook was still being used for this purpose. Legal proceedings were brought in 1867 but failed to achieve anything. It wasn't until the late 1870s that Hanley constructed a sewage-disposal works in Leek Road on the site of Trent Hay farm. Pollution of the Trent and the Fowlea Brook remained a problem. Privies, by 1883 had still not been replaced by water-closets.

There were no public baths yet. The Eastwood Mill Company had opened baths for swimming and private baths, in 1849. So, a couple more years to wait for that. Hanley also had to wait for the medical baths in Slack's Lane, and the public swimming bath, with private baths attached. These were near Macaroni Bridge on the Trent and Mersey Canal, about a quarter of a mile north of Etruria. These wouldn't be built until 1851 and 1854 respectfully.

These had closed soon after 1858 and, by 1873, were in Lichfield Street.

On our walk I also noticed the 'house of recovery' for the poor, was still there. I told John what I knew about the place – that it had a dispensary and a reception ward, supported by voluntary contributions. It had been built around 1803-4 at Etruria Vale, north of the Bedford Street canal bridge. It was a brick building, three stories high. It hadn't been sufficient, even with extensions and a new two-story building, known as the North Staffordshire Infirmary, designed by Joseph Potter of Lichfield, had been erected around 1815-19 on 6 acres of land called Wood Hills, on the east side of Etruria Vale Road, opposite the site of what later became Etruria Park. Fever wards had been added between 1828-9 largely with the proceeds of a bazaar held at Newcastle, and wards for burns in 1852.

John, had been listening to me and my memories and, speaking from his sick bed, informed me that a north wing had been built in 1855 with money given by Charles Keeling of the White House, Newcastle. The old infirmary building stayed until it was purchased in 1867 by the British Gaslight Company. The infirmary was moved in 1869 to Hartshill, owing to the danger of subsidence following development of the ironworks and coal mines near the second building.

"There was a fire brigade as well on that walk - something I hadn't noticed before." John explained that this was set up in 1853.

"Strange that Hanley had a fire brigade but no proper police force. I would have thought the two would have gone hand in hand, John?"

John, who seemed to know all this information, and dates, advised me that Hanley didn't get a borough police force until 1870. "Selly suds", he came out with and laughed. He explained that they couldn't pay for or get enough people to man the police force and members of the fire brigade had to act as special constables, when required. "Codna run a knaze-op in a brewery". He added that Wedgwood was the man who knew what was what and set up a private brigade of a captain, 10 men and one fire engine at his factory.

It was good to hear John laugh. Maybe the ice had been broken. It was a subject John was interested in, so I just carried on talking. "What was pleasing to note, John, was that most of the streets in Hanley and Shelton, had been tarred and the pavements were paved with blue brick." John said this had been accomplished in 1849.

"This was so much better and cleaner than the mud roads that were there before. Ladies with their long dresses could actually walk around without having to lift their skirts while crossing puddles of mud, or get mud-splattered by passing horse and carts."

John added that the control of the highways passed under the control of the borough council as the Hanley Local Board under the Act of 1858. He also stated that it wasn't until 1879 that this board finally declared Hope Street, Stafford Street, Trinity Street, Brunswick Street, Piccadilly, Clough Street and Sun Street as main roads, and thus took responsibility for their upkeep.

"Anyway, John, we finally got to the big field in Etruria. When Ricardo arrived, there was a huge surge towards the roped-off area and we were being pushed and shoved all over the place. People just wanted to see what was happening and to get to the front.

Unfortunately, poor Ricardo got pushed and shoved in the stampede as well."

"Yer, it wosna 'is dee. Efter 'e geeve 'is spaych, it wus tahm fer 'im te do 'is foncy bet en deg into th'earth te cut the fost sod. Frum wut ah cod seey, 'is speede wus silver in culour, med special-loik fer th'ceremony, not a prupper deggin' tooel. Trobble wus, eet 'ad ben so darn dray, thut the speede actually boockled 'neath 'im,.... than a gust o' wind gor up, en 'is 'at blooe aff."

"There were oohs and ahs in the crowd but we just thought it was funny, not meant to be, but we couldn't help but laugh."

John laughed at this and I giggled remembering the occasion. I didn't know if John was just putting on a show – making the best of a bad thing as he wasn't well enough to walk out under his own steam, but still keeping very wary of me. He had laughed, but it was a sort of false laugh. I got the underlying impression that he was probably thinking that he had survived so far, and I hadn't poisoned him or bewitched him, so just go with the flow. So, my giggle was cut short. I had a long way to go to try to get him to trust me again. He was just trying to build up his strength so he could walk away. It was a shame.

"Bucknall en Northwood station wus a beet of a tarm coming efter thut, but we got it." John added, also obviously seeing my disappointment.

I carried on. "Yes, unfortunately, we were no longer together then. We'd had Geoffrey, but I don't want talk about that at present. I want to remember good things.

"It was 1864, I believe. Geraldine had been born in 1850 and her 14th birthday was coming up. She was becoming a young lady now. She'd left school at 12 and was helping me on my rounds as a nurse. I thought she needed cheering up a bit, something to get her out, be a part of what was happening around her. Hearing about the opening of the station, I thought it would be nice to take her on a short trip to Leek." I was looking forward to it myself as I'd loved travelling on the steam trains on various holidays that I'd taken in my former life. These trains had been meticulously restored back to their former glory and most of the people who worked them were volunteers, such people who had loved the trains in their youth until they'd been axed. Of course, it had been years since I'd travelled on a steam train, or any train come to that, and to be travelling on one of the original trains at near enough the start of steam train transport, would be wonderful. "Geraldine was excited at the prospect, but she wondered if you could come along too."

....

I was remembering that conversation. **Geraldine had been saying:**

"I know dad's interested in the development of the railway. I've seen him around and we have had a few chats." She added, more as a mutter than anything, "It's such a shame you two split up." - but I did hear her.

"Now, Geraldine, you know your dad and I aren't going to get back together. It's been too many years and too much bad feeling. When you've spoken to him, has he ever mentioned me?"

"No, mum. I tell him how you're getting on, but he doesn't respond, just changes the subject.... - he'd ask me how I was doing at school or something similar."

"See, there's no way he'll come along and he definitely wouldn't listen to me if I asked him, but, if you've really got your heart set on him coming along, next time you see him, try asking him yourself. I don't hold out much hope though, so don't come back disappointed and crying."

......

"Anyway, John, I don't know what she said to persuade you, but she must have begged and pleaded and finally you agreed, albeit reluctantly. I didn't know what to expect. I didn't even know if you'd talk to me, just ignore me and talk to Geraldine."

"Yer, ah codna let 'er dine. Way'd mack do, sum'iw or t'uther."

CHAPTER 10 – THE TRAIN RIDE

"So, Geraldine arranged to meet you at the station, John. It was quite a long walk there for us, as you know, and really a long way round to get to Leek, from here, but we all wanted to ride on the train. You were a bit sombre when we met, grunted a hello, but greeted Geraldine heartily, which was nice."

"Yer, ah dinna know whut te say te yer. It 'ad bin so lung sin we'd sayn aych uther."

"You'd even bought her a present for her birthday. A book about trains, I believe. She seemed quite happy with it, not necessarily that it was about trains, but that it was something that you had personally got for her."

"Ah dinna no whut te git 'er, raylly. Ah've not 'ad much te do wi' yong lesses."

"Nevermind, I'm sure she loved it."

"Anyway, we looked around while waiting for the train. There were just two tracks, for a train coming from Leek and a train coming from Stoke. There was a wooden waiting room on our side, with an apex slate-tiled roof, and a smaller waiting room over the other side followed by a row of little shacks, possibly for offices or storage. One train arrived, but this was a goods train carrying big wagon-loads of flint, presumably for the mill at Bucknall. Horse-drawn carts were backed up to the wagons, for this flint to be loaded onto, and men and boys were up the top throwing the flints into the carts. It looked like really heavy work as men and boys were sweating and puffing. There was a man standing by, who turned out to be a foreman. We enquired about the load and he told us that the flint would be taken to the burning kilns, loaded up between layers of slack to burn the flint and break it up. This would then be ground to powder for making pots."

....

Our train finally arrived. It had a huge, black steel engine, belching smoke, with huge metal wheels that were turned by a complicated system of shanks and pulleys – a true feat of engineering! The train driver was in an open-sided cabin and I could see a coal stoker bearing a spade. Behind this cabin was a wagon full of coal. It was a remarkable sight for Geraldine, who had never seen anything like it. Of course, I had seen the like in various transport museums, and had been on a few steam engine rides and seen various films, such as The Railway Children, featuring these old steam trains. Of course, I couldn't mention any of this, but it brought back good 'futuristic' memories, of good times, when I had money and could take holidays. It was so good having a car, in those days, to go anywhere I wanted, visit all the museums, go on jaunts, even go abroad on high-speed electric trains. But, this was the start of the history of the train – steam power, something that would forever be fascinating. The coaches were wooden, with separate compartments that could hold about 8-10 people. The doors were opened by a metal turn handle and the windows could be raised and lowered by a leather strap. The seats were nicely padded, seat and high-padded back. It was luxury compared to riding in a horse-drawn wagon. John had bought us first class tickets. The third class was little more than wooden slat seats, open to the elements, immediately behind the coal wagon, and the poor passengers, in this carriage, had the smoke from the chimney blowing in their faces, choking them, with bits of cinder alighting on their clothes. These passengers were huddled up with their backs to the engine, holding hands and scarfs over their faces for protection.

We had to step up onto a metal step to get into the carriage and I found John at my side, giving me a helping hand.

"Thank you John." I proffered. "That's very kind of you." It felt good to have his solid arm supporting me.

The station master, looking dapper in his uniform, dropped his white flag and the train started off with a chug, chug, and the whistle blew, then a flume of white smoke blew past the window. I was excited and John was smiling. Geraldine looked a bit wary but I told her there was nothing to worry about – just sit back and enjoy herself, or look out of the window.

The train chugged on under the main road and Finney Gardens came into sight. It was, at the time, a market garden covering 16 acres on both sides of the railway track. The plant nursery was owned by Theophilus Cartlidge who developed his nursery, having areas for picnics and serving ales and wines.

Footsteps in the Past – The Secret

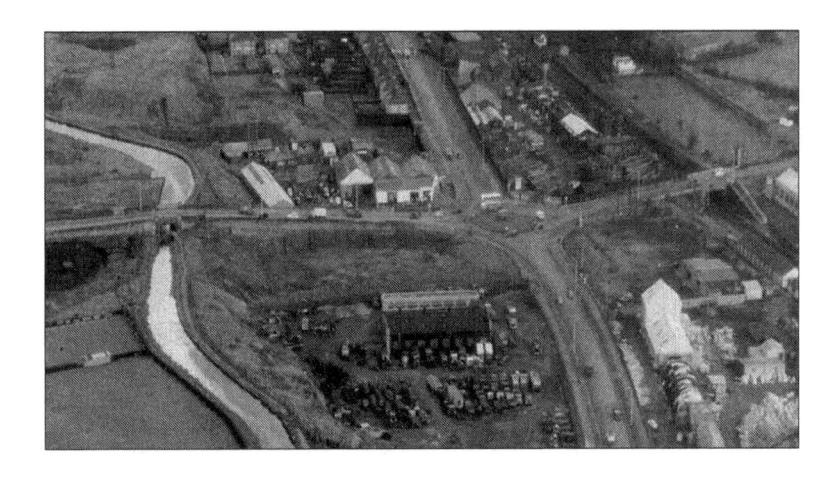

To the left is the Caldon Canal which was opened in 1779 - it joins the Trent and Mersey Canal at Etruria and was built to carry minerals from the uplands of the Peak District to the Potteries.

Bucknall Road runs left to right across the picture and it crosses the canal at the Ivy House Bridge. The roundabout is the junction of Bucknall Road and Leek Road (the section of the road nearest the camera was originally Abbey Road).

At the crossroads is a saw mill. Front left is Beeches Garage and front far right is the Bucknall Station platform.

"John, that's Finney Gardens – strange seeing it from this angle. There is always something happening there."

"Yer, ah belayve thah'd sommit just bin on. A two- dey gala en rose show, 4th and 5th July. Thah were praizes ge'en te the best competitors. En thee 'ad singers, Miss Moorland end Meesters Thurnbull, Gannon, Hall en Emery, Ef mar mimory sarves may raight. Thee also 'ad a brass and string bond wi' dancing. Ah so eet advertised int' Staffordshire Advertiser."

140

Yes, John was always good with names and remembering facts. Facts and figures just left me after a while, especially now that I was in my 60s.

"Ah wus thenkin' o' invatin' yer efter Geraldine gor in totch, but ah thowt bitter o' it."

"I would have loved to have gone with you, John. I wish you had invited me."

John changed the subject, "Thee 'ad races theer tooe - ponny reeces, waggon reeces and trotting reeces. Ah went theer fair raegular loik. Thusands o' payple used te tarn up - Ah osso wint te pegeon shooeting en ah ayvn tooek pert. Ah won sommit in '73 - a monney praize.

"Well done, John. Yes, I've seen the adverts for all sorts of sporting events and galas, athletics and walking competitions – always with prizes. There is always something going on.

......

Back to the present, I asked John if he was at Finney Gardens for the walking competition in '76 when Henry Vaughn was meant to do a 30 mile walk in five hours. "If I recall correctly, he walked for a little under two hours, after he'd done 12 miles, had a break, then carried on but couldn't complete the course. Still, he tried. Then they'd have games of prison-bars between eleven of the best runners of Longton, Fenton and Stoke and a similar number from Hanley, Burslem and Tunstall. The winners each received a silk handkerchief.

"Yer, ah wuz theer. Ah rimember eet well. A silk 'ankie's nor much o' a praize but ah supposs eet's th'onour o' wennin'."

However, John, I seem to recall something not so good that happened at Finney Gardens. It was reported in the Staffordshire Weekly Times and there was all sorts of chatter about it. I believe it was some time in 1873..... that a young girl, Caroline Flynn, about 13 years old, was found drowned in the Trent, the section that runs through Finney Gardens. I believe she worked for the owner. There was talk that she'd committed suicide. Seems she didn't turn up for work. The police dragged the river and the dragnet finally caught on something near the railway bridge, where the water is about six feet deep. They'd found her body. There was an inquest at the Trent Tavern but nothing conclusive was discovered, apart from the girl being moody and taciturn – shame that. She must have had something she was worried about. I mean, she had a job, so had money"

"Oo knars, shay coddave gor 'erself int family weey."

"Possibly, but then that would be rape. Poor thing."

....

After Finney Gardens, the train headed north to Abbey, leaving behind the smoking potteries of Hanley, in the West. However, there were still notable signs of industry along the way. At Abbey there were pipe works and an old clay pit on the right. The scenery turned into countryside - fields with cattle, sheep and horses, with rough grass close by the tracks, that wavered violently as we passed, with the disrupted air caused by the movement of the train. Geraldine was busy looking out of the window, as the train chuffed along, fascinated with the white plume of steam from the engine floating past, "Be careful not to lean too far out of the window, Geraldine, there may be another train coming in the opposite direction. She looked a bit startled and shrank back into her seat. To allay any possible fears I said, "Geraldine, do you remember that poem I taught you – about the train – From a Railway Carriage? This train just reminded me of that poem, the poem just chugs along to the same rhythm as this train, and so apt as here we are looking out of a railway carriage." It was a poem I had been taught at school in 20th century. I had told Geraldine that I had made up the poem myself. I couldn't possibly tell her it was by Robert Louis Stevenson, as he was only born the same year as Geraldine, 1850, so would have been 14 as well at this time. I recounted the poem.

> Faster than fairies, faster than witches,
> Bridges and houses, hedges and ditches;
> And charging along like troops in a battle
> All through the meadows the horses and cattle
> All of the sighs of the hill and the plain
> Fly as thick as driving rain;
> And ever again, in the wink of an eye,
> Painted stations whistle by.
>
> Here is a child who clambers and scrambles,
> All by himself and gathering brambles;
> Here is a tramp who stands and gazes;
> And there is the green for stringing the daisies!
> Here is a cart run away in the road
> Lumping along with man and load;

And here is a mill and there is a river:
Each a glimpse and gone for ever!

Geraldine joined in with me for the last couple of lines, bumping herself up and down on the seat in semblance to the rhythm of the poem and the train. We both had a giggle afterwards.

We were passing a colliery on the right now – possibly Mossfield, then a corn mill. The Trent and Mersey canal was following the track on the right, or should I say the track followed the canal. There was another colliery coming up on the left, then we arrived at Milton Junction. There was a signal box here, a two-storey brick-built little construction, with windows all round on first floor level and a tiled apex roof, but the ground floor was totally brick, with no windows. There were stairs going up on the outside to the first storey. I saw someone come out and hand something to the driver. John explained that this was a single-line token. It seems that Milton Junction was not really a junction but was the intermediate point for two single line sections between Leekbrook and Stoke. The Milton to Leekbrook section was operated by token, released from the token apparatus interlocked to each signal box. What I gathered from that was that trains to and from Stoke at this section would now be running on the same single line of track. That was a bit worrying. "What if another train comes from Leekbrook towards us?"

"Ne'er feayre. Thut's wut tockens 'r fer. Onnly one treen con pass on thus stritch o' laine at a tarm. Eet wonna 'appen."

A bit relieved, I carried on looking out of the window. The line seemed to be swerving towards the east. We passed Foxley Bridge with its brick works. We seemed to have lost the canal. We went over a bridge and I saw the canal appear again on the right hand side. The train then stopped again. This was Stockton Brook Station. The railway line seemed to pass diagonally under a crossroads. It appeared to be a busy main junction, presumably part of the Leek Road. I could just make out the Hollybush public house. Then we were travelling over Stanley Moor, past the flint mill there. We'd lost the canal. There appeared to be another bridge up ahead. John pointed out that this was in fact a section of the Caldon Canal passing over us, in an aqueduct, at a height of 490ft above sea level. He informed us it was built by James Brindley in 1777 and is believed to be the highest canal in Britain.

The next stop was Endon and we got the Trent appearing again on the right. This was, what John pointed out, a canal feeder, on the left. We then passed through Wall Grange Station and the large expanse of Hollinghay Wood. We then entered Cheddleton Junction. I remember thinking that this was a long way round to get to Cheddleton – I could have walked to Cheddleton, had I a mind to. The station here was more like a house, set back quite a walking distance from the main road. It was brick-built with tall chimney pots and a steeply-sloping slate roof. The building was intricate, built in the Jacobean style and somehow, looking, like a smaller version of Ash Hall. There were also lines running off to makeshift shelters, what John stated was a goods yard. Anyway, it was here the line turned northward. John said we were now on the Churnet Valley branch. The train then went through a tunnel, luckily just a short tunnel, as it was eerie and the sound around deadened. We all said, "Ooh" and Geraldine looked a bit startled. We carried on to Barnfield, then Leekbrook Station, where there was another signal box, in the same style as at Milton Junction. Here the single line token was exchanged again. We were back onto the two-line track and we finally arrived in Leek. On alighting from the train, I tried to work out where we actually were. There were lines running in all directions, sidings and works sheds for train repair, a signal box but no waiting rooms or refreshment rooms and no footbridge, so we dubiously and carefully had to walk over the lines to head in the direction of the main town, being much aware of movement of trains. We held onto Geraldine's hands, me on one side and John on the other.

There was a market on, which we took our time going around. It was quite bustling with folk looking for a bargain. John actually picked up a hole-maker drill for his work. It had a screw-shaped drill, which was turned by a handle. I remembered that my dad had one, when I was young, for his work as a plumber. There were some lovely tea sets but I really didn't have any money to spend, so just looked around. Geraldine picked up some ribbons, possibly to decorate her bonnet. We then headed to the Swan with Two Nicks for lunch. Fortunately, John was paying. The name of the pub derives from the centuries-old tradition of marking birds' beaks with nicks (or necks) to denote ownership. At the back, at the time, was an extension for a grocery and provision store. It is a grade ll listed timber-framed building, said to be Leek's oldest inn.
....
I remembered the Swan with Two Nicks, as The Green Dragon, just over the road from the magnificent St Edward the Confessor church.

I went there once and saw a small, framed picture of Sergeant Major John Allen, who rode in the ranks of the 13th Light Dragoons at the Charge of Balaclava on 25 October 1854. He became landlord of the pub from 1887 until his death in 1894. Of course, Balaclava was yet to happen and that little picture wasn't there. It would have been nice to have met him and hear him recount his stories. Maybe I'd get a chance to meet him, after 1887, if I was still alive. My interest in this had been enhanced, after meeting Jean and Paul Ashton from Werrington, who had collections of army costumes and memorabilia, including ladies' dresses from the 19th century. They would wear these costumes to battle re-enactments and had even gone to Waterloo for a re-enactment of the Battle of Waterloo, where they had met Frenchmen, giving orders in French and singing French war songs. They were quite fascinating and what's more, they actually owned the helmet that Sergeant Allen had worn at the Charge of the Light Brigade! I had also noticed the Lord Raglan pub, on the corner of Brook Street and Compton. Lord Raglan was the man who gave the order that resulted in Sergeant Major Allen and the rest of the 600 riding into the 'Valley of Death'.

From what I could remember from my history lessons, this was a fiasco of misunderstanding. Lord Raglan, the commander in the Crimea was looking on as a huge force of Russian infantrymen overwhelmed three of the Turkish-held earth forts. This had left the British supply port of Balaklava. A 'Thin Red-Line of Highlanders and an uphill charge by the Heavy Brigade of British horse, had stopped the Russians taking the port. Lord Raglan gave Lord Lucan orders to advance to recover the hill but Lucan wouldn't move until infantry arrived. By this time, the Russians were trying to remove the British naval guns sited in the earth forts. Raglan wrote a quick order that he wanted the cavalry to advance rapidly to the front, follow the enemy and try to prevent them from taking the guns off. What he meant by this was that he wanted Lucan to move the cavalry forward on both sides of a relatively gentle slope, and possibly even along it, to hasten the Russian withdrawal and encourage them to abandon the British guns.

However, Lucan, on reading this garbled message, was adamant he wasn't going to advance without infantry. The messenger, Nolan, then declared that Lord Raglan wanted the cavalry to attack immediately. It seems that Nolan was so contemptuous of Lucan's ability, so desperate for the cavalry to show its worth, that he failed to provide the officer with the necessary clarification. The written order had not mentioned any such attack. All Lucan could see from his position was a Russian battery of eight cannon at the end of the valley. Raglan should have taken into account the fact that Lucan's view of the battlefield was limited and should have made the final order more precise. Lucan should have insisted on clarification from Nolan, but he allowed his pride to get the better of him. So, instead, Lucan ordered the charge of the Light Brigade, led by Lord Cardigan, at this Russian battery instead of attempting to recover the captured naval guns of the Causeway Heights. At this point there was a battery in front, a battery on each flank and the ground covered with Russian riflemen. Literally a death trap. They broke through the Russian lines and, instead of capturing their guns, and making off with them, they attacked. On re-grouping it was discovered that about 100 men had been killed, about 200 wounded and 50 missing, with the death of about 400 horses.

This was a war fought after the Russian Tsar refused British and French ultimatums to withdraw his troops from Ottoman territory. Although the British kept Balaclava, their main supply route was cut and, basically, when the winter came they had no fuel, inadequate shelter and insufficient food. The British troops fell easy prey to disease, particularly cholera and typhus. The grand British army had fallen due to gross incompetence and aristocratic hauteur. By the end of the war 21,000 British soldiers had died, only a quarter from enemy action, the rest from disease and malnutrition. According to Lord Cardigan, Lucan ought to have had the moral courage to disobey the order until further instructions were issued. Raglan, Lucan and Nolan were all to blame.

Corporal Allen, as he was then, was one of the few who received the Distinguished Conduct Medal for heroism during the disastrous attack. His horse was shot from beneath him as he sped into the 'valley of death'. Allen was at the front of the attack and took a bullet in the knee in the thick of the carnage, after his horse was shot dead beneath him. As he made his way back to British lines, he found fellow trooper, Joseph Malone, trying to rescue a wounded officer. They caught a riderless horse and put the officer on it, then managed to get the casualty back to safety. Malone won the Victoria Cross. Allen had entered the battle as a Corporal and left it as Sergeant. He retired after that campaign, to Leek, in 1868 where he earned himself the post of Troop Sergeant-Major to the Leek and Biddulph Queen's Own Yeomanry. He died on 30 July 1894, aged 68 and was given full military honours at his funeral, the route from the Swan being thickly lined with people and a firing party of nearly twenty soldiers fired three rounds over his grave.

As I said, it would have been nice to have talked to him of his exploits but it seems he rarely talked about this battle, or the others in which he took part, confining his remarks to "having been one of the lucky ones". But he was the proud possessor of four medals – that for the Crimean War with Alma, Balaclava, Inkerman and Sebastopol bars bearing the 1854 date; the Turkish War Medal 1855; the D..M, and one for Long Service and Good Conduct.

....

Retreating from my reminiscences, I interrupted John and Geraldine's conversation. "I seem to remember, John, that a lot of people marched from Leek, heading towards Burslem, to get involved in the Pottery riots back in 1842. That was a horrible day, 16th August. I was scared out of my life. Something I'll never forget."

"Yer, them war deastrous deeys. Ah'll nivver fergit 'em missel, en you baying puorly bed efterwods."

"Yes, we were cowering behind the wall of the Big House, the Wedgewood House, in Burslem, as the army came riding up, and Colonel Powys was reading the riot act to the starving thousands who had descended on the town and where poor Josiah Heapy, that unfortunate young man, got shot by the army. Didn't we hear that the poor lad came from Leek?"

During our conversation, there was a gentleman on a table nearby, who had presumably been listening. He got up and introduced himself.

"Sorry, to interrupt you. I am Mr Edwards. I have been listening to your talk about the Pottery Riots. I'm a bit of an historian and was here when the Pottery riots took place. Maybe I can throw a light on what was happening here during that time."

"By all means, Mr Edwards. We would love to get a better understanding of how Leek was involved. We are Mr and Mrs Wood and this is our daughter, Geraldine." I didn't want to say to a complete stranger that we had been separated for so many years, it wasn't his business to know, anyhow.

"OK, of course, as everywhere, during the 1830s-40s, there was unrest. We're not potters here in Leek but there is industry, mainly silk. We've got quite a few mills, as you will see if you care to peruse the town. Anyway, the mill workers were also fighting to improve their rates of pay for piecework, and this led to at least one strike in 1834 by handloom weavers. A short-lived silk operatives' union had been formed by May that year when over 400 men and women marched through the town with considerable ceremony, waving banners and placards, at the funeral of a fellow member. However, the mills hands struck again, against another pay cut, in 1838."

"Yes", I interrupted. The potters and miners had had their pay cut numerous times and found themselves on the breadline, starving, with nothing to look forward to but the workhouse, and we'd followed the preachings by various Chartist speakers, attempting to get their People's Charter approved by Parliament and to get their pay rate brought back to previous rates before the cuts."

"Quite true. You're well informed. A government commissioner who came to Leek later that year and John Richards, a Chartist missionary, who formed a political union in the town in 1839, found many of the hands poverty-stricken and resentful. In January 1842, the Leek branch of the Anti-Corn Law league sponsored a petition to Queen Victoria from the women of Leek, that drew attention to working-class distress in the town.

Leek became involved in the Chartist unrest later in 1842. On Saturday, 13th August, groups of young men arrived in the town, claiming to be strikers from neighbouring manufacturing towns, and they went round begging at houses. The following day, the Leek magistrates were warned that several thousand men, who were occupying Congleton, were preparing to march on Leek. The magistrates swore in at least 350 special constables and sent to the Potteries for troops. They seem also to have organised a mounted patrol of the parish. On the morning of 15th August, the Newcastle and pottery troop of yeomanry cavalry arrived. Young men and boys, armed with bludgeons, were already drifting into the town from the direction of Congleton, but the main body of marchers, variously estimated at 2,000 and 4,000 men, did not arrive until 11am. They were mainly from Congleton and Macclesfield, with a few from Stockport and Manchester.

Preceded by a band, they marched into the market place, where they were confronted by the magistrates, the yeomanry, and the specials. There was a brief altercation, but when the marchers assured the magistrates that no violence was intended, they were allowed to pass. Some begged through the town in groups for food and money. Others went round the silk mills and dye works, forcing those, that had not already been closed by a strike, to shut. The marchers then went to the cattle market for a meeting at which their leaders called on the Leek workers present to join a general strike. In the afternoon, most of the marchers returned to Congleton, but some remained to organise a march on the Potteries the following day, 16th August. They slept in a plantation on the Ball Haye estate and were fed by local sympathisers. As you know, there were riots in the Potteries on 15th August, and on the 16th the Newcastle and Pottery yeomanry returned from Leek before dawn to restore order. A few hours later the marchers who had remained at Leek overnight, set off for the Potteries, accompanied by a large number of Leek workers. A troop of dragoons had already been called out to deal with looting in Burslem, and a magistrate, receiving news of the approach of the Leek and Congleton men, read the Riot Act."

"Yes, I interrupted, we were there. It was Colonel Powys reading the Riot Act. John and I were hiding behind the wall at the Big House in Burslem. We saw the marchers arriving, carrying stones and coshes and the like. One of them called out to Colonel Powys, after he read the Riot Act, telling the mob to go home peacefully, saying 'What have we got to go home to?', They needed food, they were starving. They'd rather die fighting for their rights. Then the mob began to throw stones at the dragoons, who opened fire. One dragoon saw Josiah Heapy, a 19-year old shoemaker, who was standing by the wall of the Big House, pick up a stone, and he turned his rifle on him and fired, killing him outright. Several people were wounded. The dragoons then charged the crowd and dispersed it."

"Yes, I was there in that mob. It was a fearsome display, people running for their lives, scattering through and in and out of the Shambles. I got back safely to Leek, thankfully and, later that day, the leading inhabitants of Leek, fearing that their town would again be overrun, sent urgent appeals to the authorities for troops. But, they'd obviously listened to the woes and tribulations of the starving masses and, in the evening, they handed out a large amount of bread to the poor. The next day, 17th August, the district army commander agreed to send a company of the 34th Regiment of foot and also the Lichfield troop of yeomanry, which was in Newcastle. The yeomanry may have reached Leek the same day; the infantry arrived early on 18th. Heapy's funeral at St Edward's later that day, apparently led to no disorder, and the silk masters and dyers reopened their works the following morning. The troops were still at Leek on 20th August, but there seem to have been no further disturbances.

As you know, there was finally a breakthrough after all of these strikes and marches and on 6th September the United Branches of Operative Potters was formed. Soon after that The Cotton Spinners Association and National societies were formed for the printing trades and Tailors and Shoemakers, plus Operative Stonemasons, United Flint Glass Makers' Society, Miners' association of Great Britain and Ireland."

"Thank you for that, Mr Edwards, that has been most enlightening." and we bid Mr Edwards goodbye, to have a walk around Leek.

Leek had changed from a quiet market town to a silk-weaving centre, with several large mills, one of which being Brough, Nicholson & Hall plus the Big Mill off Mill Street, The Wellington Mills on Strangman Street, Compton Mills on Compton Street, and California Mill off Union Street to name a few. Textiles and dyeing were a fundamental part of the town's livelihood and it had gained national fame for its embroideries, buttons, ribbons and sewing silks and attracted many artists and designers, including William Morris. I noticed there was a workhouse on Brook Street, which sent shivers down my back, plus Ash alms houses on the corner of Broad Street and Compton Street. The Leek Philharmonic Society had been established in 1839 by Benjamin Barlow, who was appointed choirmaster and organist at St. Edward's church. It seems he used to give concerts, held in the Assembly Room at the Green Dragon. There was also a cattle market every alternate Wednesday. Luckily, it wasn't happening while we were there. I could imagine the mayhem of cattle being driven through the narrow, cobbled streets and the stench of sweating cows and cowpats. They would be driven into pens sited in an open space at the east end of Derby Street, where they would be exhibited for bids taken at auction for their purchase.

Talking about mayhem, we noticed that virtually every other place in the centre was selling beer. There were even people who had opened the front rooms of their homes to the public for the purchase and drinking of beer, plus quite a few brothels and gambling dens, places that had their windows blocked up, but were actually 'speak-easies', where anything could go on behind closed doors. These venues were, naturally, frequented by some customers having one too many, and, on entering the fresh air, were seen reeling around trying. Failing to walk in a straight line, not helped by the cobbles, they resembled the term 'land lubbers', brought into use by sailors coming ashore and trying to find their stability after being on board for long stints. Of course, Hanley and any town centre was the same, loads of little establishments selling beer, now turned into brothels and places where criminals would hang out. This was the result of the government introducing the Beer House Act in 1830, which was an attempt to stop the sale of spirits. This law meant the sale of gin, or other spirits made from grain, was forbidden but people were allowed to brew at home. As a result, licences were issued willy-nilly and the number of pubs in places like Leek rocketed. Over the years, however, many had disintegrated into venues for low life. I was glad that John was with me, and Geraldine, and that he wasn't a drinker as such. He liked one or two pints, but he needed to be in control and was always wary and protective. His work was his livelihood and, if he lost that, he had nothing. He was brought up with good work ethics, so out of the ordinary in this this day and time when so many people wanted to waste their money on drink and work when they felt like it.

Apart from the speak-easies, there were quite a few old pubs around, The Red Lion In Market Place, The Black's Head Inn on Stanley Street. Leek also had gas lighting – the Leek Gas Light Co had been opened in 1837 on Newcastle Road.

As we were walking around, John recounted the Jacobite history of Leek. It seems that, in 1715, several people in Leek declared for the Pretender, and the mob damaged the Presbyterian meeting house, but these Jacobite sympathies had declined by 1745 when Prince Charles Edward and his army passed through Leek on their way to Derby and again on their retreat north. On 3rd December a detachment under Lord George Murray passed through Leek on its way to Ashbourne. The main force with the prince arrived in Leek later the same day and took up quarters there, the prince staying at the house of Williams Mills, a lawyer, (now the Foxlowe). The Quaker meeting house, on Church Street (just round the corner to the Swan) was broken into and used as a stable. The troops began to leave for Ashbourne and Derby in the small hours of the 4th. Some remained behind and tried to seize the horses of people coming to the market; two of the soldiers were arrested and sent to Stafford gaol. The Prince, retreating from Derby, was back in Leek on 7th December. The vanguard of his army went on to Macclesfield and the rest followed on 8th. The houses of the principal inhabitants of Leek were reported as 'totally stripped and plundered', apparently in revenge for the arrest of the two horse thieves. The Duke of Cumberland passed through Leek with the pursuing force on 10th and was entertained in the market place.

So, finishing our tour, we then made our way back to the station and home.

CHAPTER 11 – CELLARHEAD

It was a lovely day, so I helped John out to the little garden I had at the back of the cottage, brought some chairs out and we sat in the sun for a while. I had my herbal garden all around us, with some under glass, waiting to be planted out. It saved me going for miles, looking for herbs to be used on my patients. I'd dug up the plants I wanted and transported them here. Some needed sandy, rough ground, so I'd made a rockery and planted them there.

"That was a good day out. I believe we all enjoyed ourselves. I'm glad, John, that you agreed to let me come along."

"Yer, Jane. Eet wus a gooed deey. Thenkin' o' thut deey remainds may o' uther gooed tarms way 'ad. Dost rimember the tarms way went te Cellerhead fer the feeres?"

"Yes, they were good and still are – held twice a year in May and November. There are four pubs there, one on each corner. I don't know how they survive as there's not much in the way of housing there, fields and farms and a couple of brickworks, one at Withystakes and the other on Hands Farm. No-one knows where the hamlet got its name though some claim it is connected with a huge cellar attached to the Hope and Anchor Inn. Others attribute it to a miserly old woman, who husband used to say of her that she would 'sell 'er yed' if it were loose!" We both laughed at that. "I believe the other pubs are the Spotted Cow, and the Red Lion with a shop, and on the diametrically opposite corner is the Royal Oak."

"Yer, the fayres are maynley for t'sale o' ''orses en kine. Thah gits a gooed gathering on fayre deeys. But, yer wrang abite 'em not macking a leeving as overy Mondeey thayse pubs'r crided en the rodds packed wi' fermers, butchers, daylers, colliers en ol en sundry, coming fer far en neer te compate in or watch sporting ivents o' ol kaynds. O' cowse, thah's a lot of booeze necked en ah've sin a few faytes. Rimember ah tock yer one Mondeey en theer were whaylbarrow reeces en the loik."

"Oh, yes, I remember now, don't know how I could have forgotten, just so many years ago, I suppose. Yes, some of the races were just ridiculously funny to watch. There was a foot race – the Moorville Mile and the six and a half miles walk to Leek too. That wheelbarrow race was hilarious with the competitors running with their barrows via Withystakes, Rownall to Wetley Rocks and back along the main road. A pretty stiff course. Oh, yes, and do you remember the mangle race? The competitors pulled or pushed an ordinary four-wheeled household mangle the good mile to Wetley Rocks. Some of these fellers were so strong. There were even handicaps in some of the races, which meant the runners ran backwards – they were tripping over themselves some of them but quickly getting up again and carrying on. We were all cheering and clapping with whooping calls if they fell."

"Yer, way tooek the two lads en trayted 'em te rhubarb depped in sugar. Way both wet oor whistles whale wutching the wristling."

"Oh yes, such nasty tactics, no rules barred, each man was all out to win, throwing their competitors to the floor and jumping on top, strangle holds, half Nelsons, and all sorts. I wasn't particularly squeamish, being a nurse, but was wondering if my assistance would be needed afterwards, to treat their cuts and bruises. I was amazed there weren't broken bones to treat.

There was so much else going on, too much to see everything – dog races pony races, even cock fighting."

"Yer, en pegeon shooeting. Yer noss ah loik the shooeting, en ah 'ad a go. Dinna wen onything thut deey though – tuthers were tooe gooed."

"We caught a bit of the bare-fist fighting. I believe there was a young man, only about 5ft 3inches, but a fine figure of a man, very neat and obviously proud of his personal appearance. He was the Potteries champion jumping. Then there was the jumping course. A series of hurdles had been put in place over about 100 yard course in five rows. The jumpers had to jump over them all, without knocking them down and then run to the finishing line. There were qualification rounds, leading to the final. There was one young man, just looked like he was flying – jumped all the hurdles with ease. Of course, he won.

Then you had a go at that machine, John – what was it called?. You know, the one where you had to hammer down on the base of the machine and a marker would be sent skywards to a bell at the top. Your hammer had to be brought down hard enough to send the marker up to ring the bell."

"Yer, en ah won sommit – som surt o' tiy."

"Yes, a sort of wooden jointed horse, with each joint threaded through with string. It was very floppy but, by holding and moving the strings from above, you could get the horse to move. The lads both had fun with that, although they both wanted to have a go at the same time and ended up fighting with the result that the toy got broken. That was the end of that!"

"Theer wuz a geezer daying weight-lefting. 'E cleemed te bay t'strungest mon in Staffordshire. 'e could left two 90lb weeghts o'er 'is yed en knuck 'em togither furteen tarms! 'E wus introduced as 'aving woked the twenty-one mayles te the Cot en Feddle Inn 'tween Macclesfield en Buxton, fer the contest. Theer wus anuther frum Yorkshire – the Yorkshire champion, 'e wus matched agin. At one pint, the competitors 'ad te peck up a masseeve stowne bo aytch, ron wi' eet, thun leeft eet up te pleece eet atop a 5ft haygh wo. Oor mon wun, but eet wus a clowse ren theng, en fer an encore, 'e lefted up two yong leedies, aytch setting on an urm, and woked arint poddock wi' 'em. 'E wus a masseeve feller, beg en tol wi' eet, wi' moscles as 'ard as aiyon. Eet wus onnly efterwards, way funt ite thut the Yorkshiremen, dopped oor lad's bayr, te tray te torn the motch in theer feevour, but the kuntest wus o'er afore the dopp tooek effect. Thun oor lad woked the twenty-one mayles wom."

"Some guy! Oh, and by this time, they were setting up a stage for singers and musicians, for the evening. We stayed for a little while and we saw another character, Jervis Forrester, one of our local men. He'd made a reputation as a writer and singer of ballads. He was introduced as having taken up composing and singing in 1838 after trying his hand as a maltster at the Hope and Anchor Inn. He'd had some of his work published in 1846 and he sang one of his ballads, 'Which is the most feasible line?' – This was a comic skit related to the various alternative routes proposed for the new railway to Cheadle."

"Of cosse, yer wotna rimember the bull reng thee 'ad theer. Thee stopped eet in 1840. Eet was sit 'twixt Methodeest Chapel and Hoppe en Anchor Inn, quate nare road. Bull beeting at the tarm wus feerly common than, as a spert. The bull wus tithered te an ayon reng set in a beeg stonne. Dogs were thin 'slipped' in, onder the direction o' masster o' ciremonies, oo way co'd the 'Bellot', en the dogs war set ont bull."

"No wonder they stopped it – that's totally barbaric. The bull had no chance – it couldn't get away or charge at the dogs, as it was tethered. That's even worse than the bull fights in Spain, I mean that's a dance and display by the toreador and he could well get gored by the bull."

"Yer, yer 'atna 'eerd the woss. Somtarms, bull wod git looese"
"No!"

"Yer, e'd ron 'avoc, aggraveeted as 'e war, en in peen, cherging at avveratheng en avveraone thut gut in 'is weey, ayven gitting ite

Footsteps in the Past – The Secret

inte meen rowd. Ah've sin it missel. Way'd o 'ad te jomp fer eet en weet 'til bull 'ad com te a stop en calmed dine, afore the owner cod fang eet en lade it beck te faild.

En tokking abite kine, well... kiyes te bay prisaise. Dunno ef yer wus theer the deey o' the ruckus wi' Mr Willshaw. Eet wus reening cots en dugs. Onyweeys, Wilshaw bowt a kiye et Cellar'ead, but the mon 'e bowt eet frum 'ad sold eet twoice. The mon oo sold it 'ad desappaired bay thun. Thee fowt fer eet en the fate wint on til thee codna stond na mer. Thee both gor pneumonia en Wilshaw dayed."

"Good heavens! Oh well, John, time for tea. You sit there a while and I'll heat something up. Afterwards, I was wondering, if you could see if you're up to climbing the stairs. If you feel strong enough I could get a couple of the neighbours to help move your bed upstairs. Don't worry if you don't feel up to it, but I just thought you might be more comfortable."

"Yer, Jane. Ah con say thut yer've bin steeying up wi' may o nait, int cheer, sin yer brote may 'ere, en thut's rate graderley, but yer no bin gitting ony proper slayp yersen. Eet's no' raight, so ah'll di mar bist. Ah'm fayling a mite better, so ah'll gi' it a tray.

CHAPTER 12 – JOB MEIGH ESTATE

It was the best night's sleep I'd had since the disaster and I bought John home. I had been so worried about John that I'd only dozed, sitting upright in the armchair, beside his bed. John had managed to get himself upstairs and so I arranged for a couple of lads to move the bed back upstairs. His single bed and mine were in the same room now.

We'd talked a little before going to sleep. Mainly about what work John had been doing since we separated.

John had still been working for Job Meigh II, up until Job's death in 1862, he then continued to work for Job and Elizabeth's son, William Mellor Meigh I. Job Meigh built his property Ash Hall, in 1837, from the profits of his pottery. It was a huge estate and in a strategic location as the Bridle Path that ran alongside the hall, was the route of coal carts from Hanley Hayes Colliery to the Hanley-Cheadle Turnpike Road. The fields over the back of the hall had coal seams, reflected in the names of the fields, "Coal Pit Field and "Slack Pit Field", and Job Meigh got a good living from the exploitation of the coal therein. This helped to pay for the construction of the estate buildings and enlargement of the estate.

> "VALUABLE ESTATE, WITH COAL MINES, &c., IN THE PARISH OF STOKE-UPON-TRENT.
> TO BE SOLD BY AUCTION BY MR ADAM WALTERS
> All that DWELLING-HOUSE, called Mettle House, with all necessary Outbuildings and Appurtenances, and about 49 acres 1 rood 32 perches of Arable, Meadow, and Pasture LAND thereto belonging, situate near the Turnpike Road, between Bucknall and Werrington, and in the parish of Stoke-upon-Trent; which said house and lands are now in the possession of Mrs Ellen Bentley.
>
> The above property has strong claims to attention. Few opportunities can occur of investing capital to greater advantage, as the estate abounds in coal of most excellent quality, which, from the vicinity of the estate to the Potteries, will always meet with ready sale. The Land is of good quality, and lies in a ring fence. The tenant will show the premises; and any further information may be obtained at the Office of Mr YOUNG, Solicitor, Lane-End."

The first property Job Meigh purchased was Metal House Farm.

It seemed also, before I arrived, the Metal House Estate had been advertised for sale at the King Head Inn in Shelton. The advert appeared in the Staffordshire Advertiser on 1st October 1836

Metal House Farm

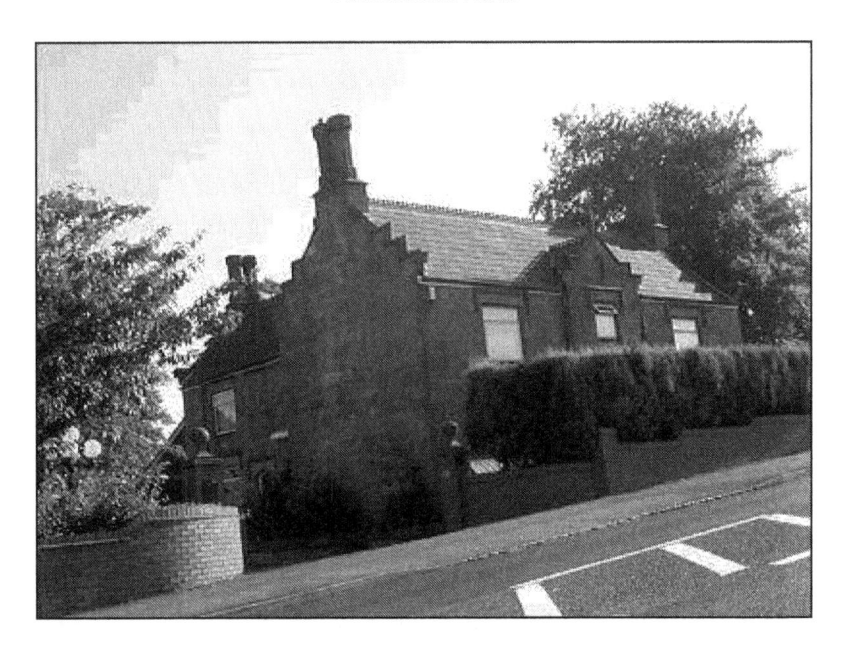

So, now Job Meigh had his supply of coal and his estate could start to grow.

"O' coss, ah've slouwed dine neow. Ah'm gittin' on en ah canna kape up wi' the yong lads. Sa ah lits 'em day mayst o' physical 'ard wark, wail ah've tacken o'er job o' supervaysor en planner. Ah still kayps may 'and in though."

Naturally, I thought to myself, there were no electrical tools. Everything had to be done by hand – sawing, making joints, drilling holes – and obviously took a lot more time, effort, and strength – just using hand drills, saws and screwdrivers. But there was more skill involved than just screwing two pieces of wood together –

proper joints had to be carved and crafted and stonework shaped to fit, with delicate, intricate mouldings.

John continued saying that, in 1851 Job Meigh rebuilt Ash Cottage, using local sandstone. Ash Cottage is located by the entrance to the Bridle Path and was the home of the new estate gardener, after John had left to work on Job's building work. The estate gardener, Joseph Weston lived there with his wife Hannah. He was 51 years old at the time. He'd been Job Meigh's carriage driver and groom while John was the gardener. Joseph had been responsible for the upkeep of the formal gardens around the Hall and the supply of fresh fruit and vegetables from the greenhouse and kitchen garden, which was located by the rear entrance off the Bridle Path. John had no further information as to whether he was still in post, or even still alive, as he'd be very old now. Probably William Mellor Meigh has retired him, although there were no retirement settlements, people just worked until they dropped, unless they had family to look after them. If he could no longer work, he probably would have been evicted from Ash Cottage and be on the street, unless he'd managed to save some money. Job Meigh wouldn't have gone out of his way to have someone live gratis in such a lovely cottage, but maybe William Mellor Meigh was a more sympathetic character.

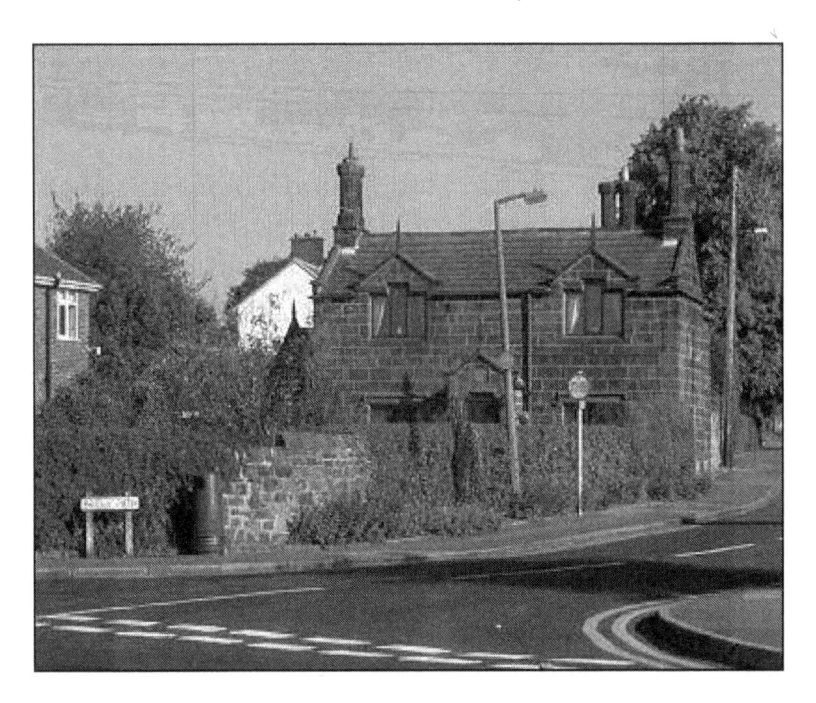

Ash Cottage

John had been involved with the demolition of the original Ash House and its replacement by the present building, constructed of local stone, the same as Ash Hall. A foundation stone recording this event stated, "This corner-stone was laid by Job and Elizabeth Meigh of Ash Hall, on the eleventh day of May 1857. Bemgno Numine." Of course, by this time, I contemplated to myself, as John was recounting this history, I was persona non gratis and not invited to the ceremony.

John was saying that William Mellor Meigh I moved across the road to Ash Hall in 1870, (he was then 63 years old) and Ash House was let to a series of tenants including John Forsythe, in

1872) and Charles Ford, a China Manufacturer, with a works in Cannon Street, Hanley. He had moved from the Hollies in Shelton.

William Mellor Meigh had been farming at Ash Farm, a grand farm of 120 acres, but gave that up in the mid 1850s and the farm was run by Ward Puckrin, a farm bailiff. Then came John Morris, a new tenant farmer, in 1862. That's when work started on the demolition of the old farmhouse and John was involved in the replacement building – a substantial two-storey, brick and tile farmhouse, quite different from the other new estate buildings, which had been built of local sandstone. "Yer, William Mellor Meigh wus quayte defferent frum 'is faither, en probably 'atna the sem amint o brass, sa 'e used breeck as it wus chayper.

Theer's somwon co'ed George Mountford in theer neow. 'E's in 'is leete 30s en 'as two min warkin' fer 'im, Charles 'Eath and William James, en 'e's got 'is waif, Anne, a yong son, George, en 'is widowed mother-in-law leeving wi' 'im."

I recalled that you could still see the Ash Farm outbuildings if you go through the car park to the back of the Ashbank Hotel that's over the Ash Bank Road from the entrance and Lodge House of Ash Hall.

"I didn't have much to do with William Mellor Meigh, John. I know he was married and had children, one of whom was in my class that I ran at Ash Hall. I believe it was Gertrude, who would have been about 8 at the time."

"Hmm, ah belayve thee 'ad siven childer betwixst 'em, en thray sarvents. One of 'em was called Ann Chetwynd, so she must have been related to Dinah Chetwynd, yer rimember 'er dosna?"

"Yes, the cook at Ash Hall. Unforgettable. She was a lovely lady, and would do anything for you. She stayed there for at least ten years, but I think she'd finally taken enough of Job Meigh's temper. She was a heroine for having stayed there that long. I suppose, because she was no longer young, he didn't try to take advantage of her, which was one good thing, but he'd scream and shout and throw things. Many a time a freshly prepared meal would be thrown across the room for Dinah to clean up, and he could be handy with his fists as well, so best to keep out of his way, when he was in one of his moods. Anyway, I believe she met a nice middle-aged widower and went to live in Stone. But, I digress; you were talking about William Mellor Meigh."

"Yer, 'e was an o'raight kaind o' mon. A beet gruff, but as leng as yer deed yer wark, 'e wus fane wi' yer. 'Es nowt lake 'is faither. 'E con control 'is timper. Yer nivver kneuw war yer war wi' Job Meigh, up one moment, dine the nixt, wi' fets o' reege. Yer knows yersen, Jane, whut 'e cod bay loik."

"Yes, I'm sorry to say this, but I'm glad he's gone. Elizabeth had a few years of peace without him, dying in 1870, which was a shame. You know he haunts the hall, don't you? It was some time after the funeral and I went to visit Elizabeth, in my nursing capacity, to see how she was. Now I don't know how much you believe in ghosts but she told me that she'd actually seen the ghostly figure of Job at the top of the winding stairs. At first it was a greeny/orangey coloured film, but gradually cleared into the figure of Job Meigh. She had been scared to death, naturally, but found herself incapable of moving. She wanted to run, but couldn't, she wanted to scream out, but nothing came out. She'd tried to turn her head away, but found herself looking at him again in fear and tremor, her body shaking all over –but she couldn't keep her eyes off him. She was frightened he was going to walk down those stairs towards her and…. well, what would he do to her. She finally she managed to let out a scream. One of the servants came running, seeing her look up and pointing, followed the direction of her arm, and screamed too. She could see him too. They both stood there looking in utter astonishment. The spectre's mouth was moving, as if saying something. They both tried to ascertain what he was trying to say and it looked like he was saying, "sorry" over, and over again. Then he disappeared and Elizabeth found herself collapsed on the floor."

"Well, 'es gor a lut te bay sorry fer, thut 'un, thut's o ah con seey."

"Anyway, let's sleep now, John. I'm really tired. We'll continue your story tomorrow."

....
The next morning, while I prepared breakfast, John started talking about my ghost story.

"Ay, theer's a feuw boggert stories arint this arrea. A feuw fellers ah knows rickon theer've sin boggerts. Theer's 'posed te bay one onder bredge on the Trent at Harecastle, known as 'Kidsgrove Boggart'. Ah've nivver sin one missel, but ah'll no seey eet's fantasy, or strung drenk, or the laight pleeyin' trecks on yer as theer's bin tay money payple o' gooed character as 've sin 'em, sober, seene payple 'oldin' dine gooed jobs."

John went on to tell me the story of the Harecastle ghost.

It seems there's a ghost boat. The tunnel is only wide enough for one barge at a time, and, given the all clear to proceed, boats have attempted to go through, only to back up quickly as there was another boat heading towards them, but they wait and nothing comes out of the tunnel. They've seen a steel barrier swing across by itself, and nothing and no-one can move it. Then, all of a sudden the barrier lifts itself up again, silently and smoothly and places itself back against the wall. On risking going through, the boats have seen no sign of this ghost boat.

He then went on to tell me the story of the Burslem 'witch', Molly Leigh. She was born in 1685 and died when she was 63. Even as a baby there were strange stories such as Molly having the ability to eat crusts when she was just hours old, that she had a "dark companion" or "familiar" – a black bird that would been seen with her at all times. There were accusations of Molly turning beer and milk sour using witchcraft. What's rather unique about this story is that Molly definitely existed.

At the side of St. John's churchyard in Burslem sits Molly's grave – facing north to south in the opposite direction from all the others; buried that way by Parson Spencer to remind us all that someone he believed was a witch is laid to rest there.

"Lercal ligend seeys thut ef yer ron arint har greeve thray tarms at 'Alloween, wail chantin' 'Molly Leigh', Molly Leigh coms ite o ar greeve en cheeses em awee ite o chochyaird."

John made "ooooh", noises, and ran round me three times.

"I do not appreciate that, John. I am not a witch and never have been, so you can forget that idea."

"Aw, cosna no tack a jokk? – mebby yer are, mebby yer aint!"

So I slapped him a bit heavier than lightly on the arm, "There, that'll teach you." I said as he flinched back. "Aw, cosna no tack a jokk?" I mimicked in his own Potteries dialect. We both smiled. I wanted to give him a hug, but I felt that this had to come from him first, and he didn't, which was a bit sad.
......
Anyway, so, John wasn't actually opposed to the idea of ghosts, but I still felt I couldn't tell him my story. I couldn't tell him I'd seen the spectral figure of myself from 21st century, in Bridle Path, warning me that something tragic was going to happen to Alfred at Lillydale Pit. It was just too close to home. He already thought I was gone in the mind, muddled or even witchy. He'd just about calmed down about me retelling the story of the school incident, when I'd blurted out the two incidents from the future, which led, directly or not to Geoffrey's death. He hadn't really accepted it, but felt he could do nothing about it. Geoffrey was dead, long ago now, and we had other things to occupy our thoughts, what with the unconfirmed death of Alfred, and his own heart attack. He needed to protect himself from stress and must have seen sense to put the

thoughts of my insanity to the back of his mind. He may even be thinking that my madness could have been just a one-off event, a temporary insanity that had passed over the years, or brought on by the first trimester of pregnancy, and that I was now sane. I was hoping that anyway, so no way was I going to upset the apple cart and make him suspect that, what he saw as temporary insanity, had not passed.

"Oh well, let's let the ghosts rest, John. Tell me more about the work you have been doing. It's nice to catch up."

John carried on from last night, about the growth of the Meigh estate, saying that there was also Little Ash Farm, about 33½ acres. This had been let to Richard Shirley between about 1841 and 1862 and had 40 acres by 1861. The next tenant was Robert Stoddard. He left in 1876 when an auction took place at the farm in November of that year.

I couldn't remember seeing any buildings associated with Little Ash Farm in 21st century – there was an overgrown track, but obviously the buildings had been pulled down.

"Job Meigh 'ad a commission agent in '61, leevin' at Mettle Ise, just below Ash 'All. 'E was David King en kem frum Lancashire. 'E acted as intermediary in besiness dayels. Ah belayves 'e sold Job Meigh's pottery abroad in return fer a shayre int profees." I remembered Mettle House as now being the Wise Owl Nursery.

"In 1854 Job Meigh desayded to build a peer o' labourers cottages at corner o' Salters Leene, just o'er rowd frum Washerwall."

Footsteps in the Past – The Secret

"Yes, I remember seeing you working on those."

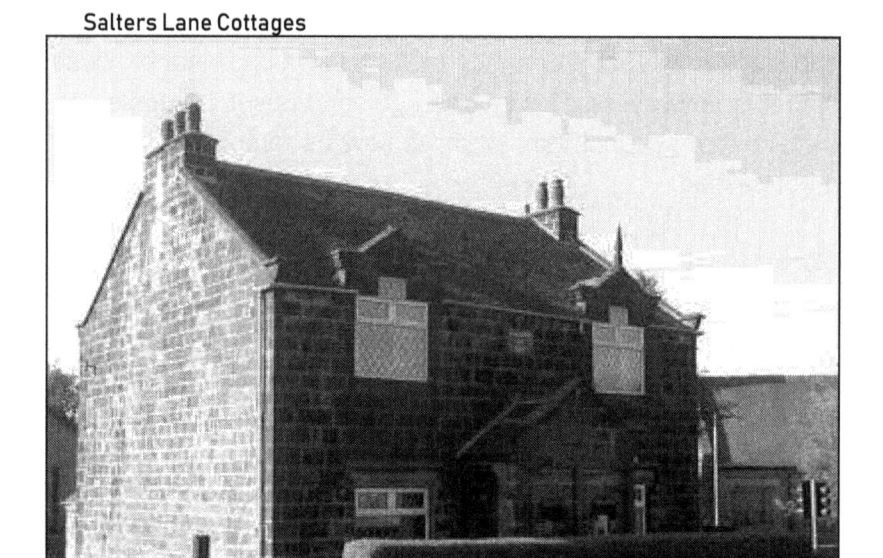

Salters Lane Cottages

"Thah war in th'old sandstone tooe, loik Ash 'All. Ah wus warking wi' William Bonnell, t'estate kerpenter, en 'e wint to leeve in one of 'em in '71, wi' 'is family. 'E mooeed frum Lawson's Ferm in Brookise Leene. Sa, 'e's leeving thah neow, wi' 'is leedy, Sarah en 'is son, Charlie, moved out some tarm ago. 'E's a cowl mainer, en 'is doter, Annie, is marrit neow. Tuther cottage es rinted bay somwon co'ed George Sillitoe – 'e's a gerdner en coms frum Leek. 'E wus theer wi' 'is leedy en foive childer. Donna 'ow thee o' fetted in as eet's onnly a smoll cottage. Thee're a beet o' a brooed, en two o' the garls canna kayp a job, donna 'ow thus George feller monages. Te mack motters woss, 'e olso 'ad som woman steeyin' wi' 'em, som tarm ago – shay wus ite o' wark tooe."

"Anyway, they look fine houses. Much better than the ones they're building around Eagle Street, on the way to Hanley. Have you seen that row of terraced houses? They're built on a slight incline and the slate roofs are built as one roof for the whole of the terrace, so the roofs rise but the windows are built on a level, straight, with some windows nearer the roof the others. It looks quite weird as the rooms inside must be shorter in height than others in the terrace."

"Yer, ah'd nivver build loik thut – eet's butched wark. Donna 'iw lang thah'll lest."

Thinking back to my previous life, I remembered seeing these buildings, and they were still going strong and occupied, so, whatever they looked like, they were sturdy enough.

"In '57 Job Meigh extinded the Lodge 'Ise bay the geete. In '61 the cowchmon thun wus German Dean en 'is leedy, theer 5-year-owd doter, en the woife's widower faither, oo wus abite 73 thun."

"That would have been a tight squeeze for that little cottage, no wonder they extended it."

CHAPTER 13 – NORTH STAFFORDSHIRE ROYAL INFIRMARY

"Sa, thut's may. Whut 've yer bin doin' yersel Jane? Ah noss yer've go' yer nursing riynds thut kayps yer bessy. 'Av yer go' yerself a manfriend? Ah noss yer goss arint wi' Dr Knight."

"Oh, don't be silly John, Dr Knight is half my age. I could be his mother."

"Just esking. Yer kaypin' yer eege well. Ah just thowght theer'd bay somwon."

"No, John. There's been no-one since you.....anyway, I've been too busy.

You probably remember that there was a smallpox outbreak in Stoke in 1871. Actually, it was all over Britain. People were dying in their thousands. Some say it was spread by the refugees coming to England to escape the French Prussian War. Anyway, Dr Knight said they desperately needed nurses at the hospital, so I agreed to help. I would walk to Bucknall to meet Dr Knight, who would drive me in his carriage to the North Staffordshire Royal Infirmary. Most times he would be able to pick me up, after his local rounds but, sometimes, there was no sign – he was probably caught up with his patients. He was actually performing operations in patients' homes. So, we made a rule that, if Dr Knight wasn't back for 8pm, I would try to get a lift from someone visiting patients

Footsteps in the Past – The Secret

and going back my way, otherwise, I would stay in a cot at the hospital. Alfred and Geraldine were all grown up by now and moved away, so there was no-one to go home to anyway."

I was thinking to myself, saying this, that there were no mobile phones or even landland phones to ring Dr Knight. - message runners wouldn't know where to find him, so that was no good either. So, if Dr Knight didn't turn up, I'd make myself as comfortable as possible – get a few hours sleep, but be on hand to be woken, should I be needed urgently.

Dr Knight was urgent that I did not stray out on my own at night, and for good reason.because there were gangs maraudering around, most notable the Rough Fleet Gang. They were not bothered about encountering any police. There was no police force in Hanley, just a locally appointed special constable. They were so powerful and so independent that no force would try to stop them and, actually, the special constable himself would not go out at night, so the criminals had right of way to do what they liked.. A couple of times one or two of them went before a magistrate and, I'd heard the gang leader, Jack Wlson, had drunk himself to death.

Right across the country, the Rough Fleet were known for their cheek and brutality. Town Road was where the Rough Fleet would wait. That was the main road between Hanley and Burslem and it was quite a dangerous road especially before the Waterloo Road was extended into Burslem. Before that there had been no direct thoroughfare. The only route from Burslem then was via Nile Street, past fields and some coal mines and everyone had to use this route. The road would turn and went up Sneyd Hill, then across into Chell Street and into Town Road, and that is where the Rough Fleet would waylay people.

They would think nothing of leaving a person disabled. They didn't intend to kill anyone, just rough them up very badly then rob them of any cash and valuables they had on them. Strangely enough though, if they did get caught, they'd try to make it up with the person by refunding and compensating. According to what I'd heard, the Rough Fleet Gang used witness intimidation, or bribary, or simply put up gang members as witnesses, in order to thwart the long arm of the law.

These gangs had started up, following the influx of people from the countryside forced to find work in the newly industrialised towns and cities. The six towns of Stoke-on-Trent, with the pottery factories, the mines and, later, the steelworks, welcomed plenty of immigrants from the surrounding villages but, while orinary people toiled away in the pits and pots, more predatory individuals had come to the realisation that a life of crime was much easier and more profitable.

There were also violent turf wars as different gangs fought each other for prominence, and to carve out their territories. Many were actually former soldiers, demobbed after the Napoleonic wars, and although trained to fight and kill, found themselves with a lack of other skills and means to earn a living, so had been terrorising towns and cities since then and, most probably their sons had followed suit, keeping it in the family.

So, I didn't try to make my own way home at night and was there on hand at the hospital to see to my patients.

"Among the biggest killers of women at this time, John, were ovarian cysts – benign tumours that, if left untreated, could crush the internal organ and stop breathing. Patients could enjoy a normal lifespan if they were removed, provided they survived the operation. Dr Knight was carrying out these operations at the patients' homes as they had far lower infection rates than on hospital wards – to avoid the deaths caused by what had become known as 'hospitalism'. I don't know if you know, John, but I've discovered that Sir Smith Child, the colleague of Job Meigh, who we met back in 1842, is currently working with Dr Spanton, surgeon at the North Staffs Infirmary, to design a detached ward for female surgical patients. Sir Smith Child is funding the building of this new ward. The plan is to have two separate bed spaces, its own staff and a strict no-visitors policy. It is due to open next year."

"Thut'll bay an emprooevement, Jane. Looeks loik eet'l seeve loives."

"That's the hope. Of course, Dr Knight has been working with the other surgeons at the hospital to ensure that all surgical areas are spotless. Surgeons have finally realised, following Florence Nightingale's lead, that, when an operation takes place, surgeons' hands, instruments and operating theatre, have to be disinfected and instruments steam-cleaned. They are to wear sterilised hats, masks and gowns and not touch anything outside of the surgery after donning this sterolised uniform and washing their hands. The death rate from post-operative shock and 'hospital gangrene' has fallen dramatically, now that operations are performed on an anaesthetized patient, in an operating theatre disinfected with carbolic, by a surgeon who had washed his hands in carbolic."

"Abite tarm". John interrupted.

I continued, "Yes, and you probably know the hospital was moved to Hartshill in 1869 from where it was before, in Etruria, as it was increasingly seen as unsuitable for patients, especially those suffering with lung infections. Can you imagine it, poor patients suffering with lung infections, trying desperately to breathe, but having only the polluted air from the pottery kilns to breathe, as the hospital was built in the middle of those chimneys belching out fumes."

Of course, I 'remembered' this hospital as the Royal Stoke University Hospital, although I'd never even visited it in the 21st century.

"Well, John. The new hospital is definitely a major improvement but, when I got there, it left a lot to be desired. It wasn't set up properly for people with infectious diseases. Patients were in wards with no separate rooms, so infections could pass easily from patient to patient. Also, this risk of infection meant that a stop had to be put on any surgery apart from that to limbs or other external parts. They were in dire straights as over half of patients operated on just died - they never recovered. The surgeons were trying various means to kill bacteria but some of these actions made the patients even worse. Would you believe they were using carbolic acid, of all things, not realising that this could be absorbed through wounds and was toxic, so the patients were dying of carbolic acid poisoning!

"Will, ah nivver." John responded.

Apart from the surgical areas, the wards were desperately in need of constant cleaning, which the nurses they'd recruited, just weren't inclined to do.. Something had to be done, but who was going to listen to me. I was just a female of the species, nothing better than a skivvy in the eyes of the surgeons and manager. There was no change there from the outside world, just a micronism of the Potteries in general - come to think of it, the world in general – the job of women was to clean and cook and bear children. We're not paid to think and have to keep our noses out of mens' business, unless, of course, we're married to someone with money or have our own money or business, then you might have a little bit of respect."

"Yer noss, ah dunna thenk thut, Jane."

"Yes, you're one of the few, the very few, John. You respect the work I do. But I've seen so much out there on my visits, with women being beaten silly, after their husbands have come home drunk from the pub, and actually being thrown out on the streets in the freezing cold, until the husband sleeps it off; wives and kiddies being starved, whilst the husband eats a hearty meal. Women actually having to sell their bodies to be able to survive, as the husband has gone off and left them with a brood of kids.

This had to change, John, and the only way to do this was, and still is, through education - but the government still doesn't believe in education for women. The general feeling before 1870, as you know, was that the uneducated masses were worthless and, as for the vote, if they ever achieved it, then the working classes would ruin the country and bring down royalty. Oh, a few have been given the vote by now, not like in the 40s, but there is still a long way to go. The Government had had to make concessions and provide schools, but children are still only being taught up to 10 years old, as of today. Before that the poor blighters would have to work. Poor, underfed, underclothed 5 or 6-year-olds in sweatshops of factories, working up to 18 hours a day, getting up at 4 in the morning, trekking to their place of work, working until possibly 10 at night, then trekking their way back home."

"Yer, ah neuw o abite thut whin ah warked int potteries afore ah met yer. Tirrible – pooer maites. But eet wus the wee of loif thin. Way neuw nay bitter, en families 'ad to sind theer childer ite te wark te arn a leeving, utherways thah codna arn enogh te fayd fomelly." John said, shaking his head.

I continued, "At work they'd regularly be beaten black and blue, by their drunken overseers, who were permanently drunk from Saturday evenings to Monday night or even Tuesday night, expecting their young staff to be doing their work in the meantime. Of course the youngsters didn't or couldn't and would get a flogging on Wednesdays as the overseers would have to put in a week's work to catch up, keeping the young beggars there until all hours with them.

This habitual drunkenness wasn't just in the Potteries, but I found this in the hospital, amongst the nurses. I would regularly find that nurses just left patients to fend for themselves, especially at mealtimes, and were not taking notes of how patients were feeling, from one day to another. They had no discipline and I was quite shocked to find them drinking alcohol together in the kitchen, drunk and unable to do their work, coming in to work when they felt like it. I was livid. Something had to be done.

Well, you've heard of Florence Nightingale, by now, John. We've read in the papers about her work in the Crimea, where she has managed to overpower the contempt of the doctors and surgeons with their ingrained views of the low status of women, by installing a military control of her nurses. She has been training them to a high degree of efficiency in nursing procedures and cleanliness, although it seems she insists on open balconies and airy wards, to counteract any hospital-generated 'miasma'. This is one of the reasons Stoke Hospital was moved away from the Potteries. Her designs are having a significant influence on hospital architecture all over Britain.

So, I went in armed with this information, ready for war, if need be."

....

What hit me on entering one of the wards, with Dr Knight, was the smell. A putrid, nauseous stink of vomit and excretia. There was a mass of beds, side by side, in this one big ward, all occupied by extremely sick and dying male patients. Looking under some of the beds, I noticed uncovered and filled chamber pots. There was a nurse there, but she was asleep at her desk – she'd obviously been there all night. Coughs and splutters were emitting from patients fighting to catch their breath, calling out for help, to the one solitary nurse, who was oblivious to their calls.

I went up to the nurse and called out to her, with no response. I then shook her by the shoulder and she opened her eyes blearily.

"Who're you?" was all I got, not a "Good morning, how can I help you?" or any courtesy, and, on getting closer, realised that her breath smelt of beer.

I introduced myself and Dr Knight, stating that we had come to assist as there was a dire need for nurses following the smallpox outbreak. I stated that we were not related, although possibly distantly. "Well, I'm nurse Elliott and I've been here all night. You'll know what needs doing, so make yourself at 'ome – I'm going 'ome." With that she got her things together and marched, rather unsteadily, out of the door. So much for a hand-over, we had been told nothing about the patients, how long they'd been there, what the diagnoses were, what medication they were on – nothing.

I gasped as she staggered away and looked, mouth open in astonishment, at Dr Knight.

"Do you know how many nurses there are? Where is the Matron? There don't seem to be any notes at the foot of the beds as to each patient's care, just a name above the bed head!"

"I know as much as you do, Jane."

We eventually found the Matron in her office, writing up copious notes on each patient, which it seemed she kept in a filing cabinet. At least she was happy to see us and introduced herself as Matron Donnelly. We explained to her the work we had been doing in the community.

"I am glad you are here, both of you. I need all the help I can get. It's a fearful mess, with nurses going off with the smallpox themselves. You'll find a few of them in the ladies' ward – some have died already. We're all worn out and stretched to our limits. The only nurses I seem to be able to get to replace them are people like nurse Elliott – who just don't want to be bothered – they're here for the pay and that's it and I haven't got the time or energy to be everywhere, overlooking what they are doing, or providing training. They know my round times and look busy enough then, but I know they're pulling the lead while my back is turned."

Dr Knight and I took a few minutes to one side to consider the situation. Tact was needed.

"Thank you, first of all, for being so candid, Matron. We can well understand the strain you are under and see you need all the assistance you can get. However, we do not feel that the situation will improve unless definite changes to the system are implemented immediately. Obviously, we appreciate the work you have been doing, and these changes will need to be approved by you, but Dr Knight and I must emphasise that patients will continue to die unless our recommendations are followed."

Matron looked a bit taken aback by this and was about to mouth something of her outrage but Dr Knight interrupted her, suggesting that an advert should be placed in the local papers immediately for anyone wishing to be trained up, adding that the advert should state that salary would be dependent on progress, hard graft, and dependability.

"Yes, Matron. There are plenty of young girls in the pottery industry, who would relish a change in occupation. They're used to hard graft and, basically, leaving one toxic situation for another, would make little difference. They're earning a pittance in the pottery kilns anyway, so, the advert should state a salary of a little above that wage to provide the incentive to change occupation. I will provide training.

"Yes," said Dr Knight, "and coming on a bit harsher than I would have done, continued, "I will be systematically checking on patients' health and medical requirements. I will expect my instructions to be followed implicitly. The first thing that I require is that patients' notes should be available at the bottom of the bed of each patient, for my reference. I will have no time or inclination to be sorting through filing cabinets."

The Matron was a little shocked at Dr Knights forebearance but acquiesced. If anyone but a doctor had spoken to her so harshly, I am sure she would have shown them the door, as she would have to me, if I hadn't been accompanied by Dr Knight.

Dr Knight added, "In my absence, I expect Nurse Knight to be treated with respect and given free rein in the teaching of the students and cleanliness of the wards. I suggest also that Nurse Knight should be given the title of Sister while in the employment of the hospital. Is that agreed?"

There was a slight hesitation in the Matron's response, but she finally agreed, stating that papers would be drawn up.

"As to the surgeons," Dr Knight continued, "leave those to me. I understand that major surgery has been suspended during this epidemic. Quite right too – the wards are in no fit state to release post-surgery patients to be infected by smallpox patients. Are there individual rooms that can be made available to house post-operative patients and those not suffering with infections?"

"Only a couple of store rooms."

"Then I suggest those store rooms are emptied immediately, cleaned, and the contents placed elsewhere. I will be speaking to the hospital manager to make funds available to have a ward partitioned off with brick walls and separate doors. Funds need to be made available otherwise, I can see this hospital, no matter how new, having to be closed as, in its present state, it is not fit for purpose."

I could see that Dr Knight was angry and he had a fight on his hands – money was always tight, but he had his contacts amongst the pottery and coalmine owners, aristocrats and benefactors, who, with a little bit of persuasion, would put up the money required. In fact, the Wedgwood family had built the original hospital. I remember Dr Knight talking about a Dr Northen, who back in 1802, was one of a group of doctors, who planned to build a clinic for the poor. He had warned that local people were in dangerously poor health, brought on by their dirty, badly-paid jobs in the pottery industry. Conditions like 'potters rot' – caused by inhaling silica dust and lead poisoning were common. Medical treatment was reserved for the rich, but for everyone else, the only choices were 'old wives' remedies and self-help books. He saw a clinic as helping the local population and arranged a meeting in July of that year, at the Swan Inn in Hanley, to consider establishing a Medical Dispensary, and a ward for the reception of fever patients. The Dispensary, which was the first public hospital in North Staffordshire – opened in Etruria in April 1804 – funded, in part, by the Wedgwood family. It gave sick patients the chance to see an Apothecary for diagnosis and treatment. It also provided vaccination against the dreaded smallpox, thanks to the pioneering work of Dr Edward Jenner. Shortly afterwards, the 11-bed House of Recovery was opened for fever patients, followed by facilities to treat general and accident patients.

Dr Knight had gone on to say that this hospital continued to expand, due to the steady flow of general illness cases, accidents in the pottery, mining and iron industries and diseases caused by lead and dust, and was moved to a bigger site in Etruria in 1819. The new hospital had a small team of support staff, including a matron and nurses and ran education programmes. It also urged coal mine and factory owners to improve their safety standards. So, this was the history of the hospital we were now standing in, in Hartshill.

I had every hope that Dr Knight would follow in Dr Northen's footsteps to be able to make the additional improvements needed here.

We left matron, Dr Knight to place the advert in the papers and I went back to the male ward to see what I could do in the meantime for the patients. Donning an apron, I started to make a start on the rigorous cleaning of the ward, emptying bed pans, cleaning up vomit and opening windows, following the instructions of Florence Nightingale. Dr Knight returned later to check the patients and give instructions to matron as to medication.

There were some really poor fellows on the ward. Smallpox was an awful disease. Luckily, I'd been inoculated against it in my former life in the 1960s. It had been one of the biggest killers in history. Its eradication in the late 1970s has been one of the greatest successes of international cooperation in public health.

I was wondering to myself why these people hadn't been inoculated as, according to Dr Knight, there were vaccinations available. Maybe they just couldn't be bothered as it wasn't compulsory for adults, or possibly they hoped there wouldn't be another outbreak. Luckily there were no children suffering with the disease as it had been made compulsory from 1853 for every child within three to four months of their birth to be inoculated. Failure to do so, would result in a £1 fine, payable to the local poor-rate.

I thought forward to the 21st century. People had been scared to inoculate their children with the MMR jab (mumps, measles and rubella) as some children, or so it was thought, became seriously affected with autism, after the injection. So, children weren't being inoculated and, what with the migration of people from other 3rd world countries - countries where there had been floods and tsunamis, war and famine, where disease had broken out and spread, diseases were now rife in countries where it was thought these diseases had been wiped out. So, what was happening now was that a great percentage of America had an epidemic of measles and thousands of people were dying.

I found out later from Dr Knight that the practice of inoculation was dangerous, and sometimes the resulting case of smallpox was severe enough to cause death. So, many were preferring to take their chances with the possibility of contacting the disease naturally, rather than risk possible death from the inoculation.

Most of the patients in the wards, male and female, were suffering with smallpox. There were others with silicosis, caused by long years working down the mines and in the pottery industry. I notificed their hands and limbs were affected with arthritis and had notable shortness of breath and weight loss, some poor things were not more than skin-covered skeletons. They were at risk of catching any other diseases, as their immune systems were so low and, in some the disease had developed into tuberculosis. There were others with broken limbs and other physical injuries. What was needed urgently was an isolation ward for the smallpox patients and others with infectious diseases, so I went about ordering the brown-coated support workers to move beds, moving non-infectious patients away from the others with smallpox, to the storage room matron had had cleared any other spare places and rooms I could find. Of necessity, until the building work had been done, it was necessary to move the male and female sufferers of smallpox into one ward, separated by curtains, so making one contagious ward.

Smallpox is a highly contagious disease, killing around 30% and leaving many of the survivors either blinded or scarred. The first symptoms are patients experiencing fever, chills, headache nausea, vomiting and severe muscle aches. After four days the fever would drop and a rash appear. The rash begins as flat or raised spots, which become raised papules. These enlarge and become filled with fluid, then pustules develop, as the fluid changes from clear to pus-like. These pustules crust over and eventually the scabs fall off after about 3-4 weeks and scarring is common. The infectious period ends only when the last scab has fallen off.

Dr Knight came to inoculate patients, although this was too late for those with the full-blown disease. The vaccination had to be given within three days of exposure, to prevent or significantly lessen, the severity of smallpox symptoms, in the vast majority of people. Vaccination four to seven days after exposure can offer some protection from the disease or may modify the severity of disease. Other than vaccination, treatment of smallpox is primarily supportive: wound care, infection control, fluid therapy, and ventilator assistance (if available).

I started making notes on patients, how they were feeling, signs and symptoms. One of my notes was on a Mr David Keeling.

29th	AM		Patient seems very restless, wandering, at times got out of bed
	PM		Very restless all day, wanting to get out of bed. No sleep. Delirium (at intervals)...
30th	AM		Patient very restless all night. Got out of bed twice; delirious at times; cough troublesome.
	PM		Has been very troublesome all day/incline to be violent... No sleep. Cough troublesome.
31st	AM		Patient very noisy until 12.30 pm. Pulse very weak at times, has been in a drowsy condition since 4am.
	PM		Very restless early part of morn, not conscious since midday.
1st			Patient died 12.50 am.

There was nothing I could have done for him apart from make him comfortable, talk to him, cold water bathing of his sores, and application of creams, keeping the area perfectly clean with disinfectants and washing bed clothing and sheets. It was so sad. Of course, he was just one of the many patients who died. Dr Knight and the doctors working in other wards at the hospital had colluded as to treatments and began to set up fluid therapy with salty water being passed to the patient intravenously, as suggested by Dr Latta. He had had great results with this therapy on cholera patients – patients he had thought were minutes away from death, being revived within a few hours, after receiving six pints of this salienated water. It was the same for patients being treated for shock or extensive skin burns.

I brought in my Lovage oils as emollients to help with the patients' breathing and added the leaves to their meals, asking the cook to add some ground seeds to the bread she baked. It wasn't much, but the oils seemed to help some of the patients.

Other doctors in the area had set up inoculation booths in the six towns to try to stem the surgance of the disease. Adverts had gone out with town cryers urging people to attend these booths, for fear of death.

An influx of young girls came to the hospital for interview, in answer to the advertisement. The Matron and I interviewed them. Most were from the Potteries. They were a fair assortment of malnourished girls, quite unkempt with some, unfortunately, suffering with wounds on their hands from the toxins in the clay, and some already with coughs. Regrettably, we had to send such girls back as we could not have anyone with open wounds on the wards or coughing over the patients. It was a shame, as such girls were the ones who needed to get out of the pottery industry. As they were young, the girls accepted had mostly had their smallpox inoculation. Those who hadn't were immediately sent to have their injection and told to come back in a few days when they felt better, advising them that the injection would make them rather unwell for a few days.

So I had my small army of nurses, who Matron managed to supply with nursing uniforms and masks. When Florence Nightingale was nursing in the 19th century, no formal uniform had been created for nurses, as modern nursing was not yet in existence. But in the years after she established the first nursing school, the nurse's uniform has evolved.

"Did you know, John, the first nurse uniforms were derived from the nun's habit, which is why they usually were a full, black, floor-length dress with a white cap and apron added. One of Florence Nightingale's first students (Miss van Rensselaer) designed the original uniform for the students at Miss Nightingale's school of nursing."

There was no reply from John, just a grunt. I don't think floor-length nurses' uniforms really interested him. So, I continued my story.

I was ready to begin my instruction to my nurses.

"You are to follow my and Matron's instructions implicity. There is to be no drinking of alcohol allowed. You are to be in the ward promptly for your shift and are to leave at the stated time and not before. This is hard work, requiring you clean and bathe each patient regularly and change the sheets. The floors are to be scrubbed each night and after any spillage or body fluids. You are to be diligent with recording patients reactions and moods, if they are eating and when and how much. These are to be recorded on the hour on the forms at the base of each bed, in good handwriting. Set tasks will be allocated on a rota basis. Matron and I will instruct you how to clean wounds and bandage. These are very poorly patients and are to be treated with dignity and respect. They are not to be manhandled roughly. If Matron or I see any of you disobeying these orders, you know where the door is, and you will not receive your pay for the week. If you notice a patient deteriorating, you are to call either of us immediately. We are here to assist you in your tasks and training, and any questions you may have. We are approachable, so please do not hesitate to contact us with any worries you may have, whatever they may be."

So, we were a team. Jobs were allocated and the ward was soon looking, and smelling clean.

Nurse Elliot had returned but was immediately allocated to another ward with a warning that she would be sacked should she be found not to be doing her work proficiently or to have been drinking during her shift.

The hospital was lucky to be able to get one of Alfred Jones' inventions to help patients with chronic breathing problems....

I didn't know what to expect as it was wheeled into the ward. Dr Latta demonstrated the machine to the team. "This negative pressure ventilation machine was invented by Alfred Jones in 1864. The patient sits inside this box with his head protruding. There's a plunger here" and he indicated a huge plunger on the left back of the machine., "This is used to decrease pressure in the box, Depresing the plunger causes inhalation, raising the plunger produces exhalation. This guage in front of the pump is the pressure guage. According to Mr Alfred Jones, this machine has been used to cure paralysis, neuralgia, seminal weakness, asthma, bronchitis and dyspepsia, and, hopefully, help our chronic patients here to breathe. There is a seat provided inside, for the patient to sit on. **Someone will have to be in control of the plunger, to operate it."**

HISTORY OF MECHANICAL VENTILATION

first American tank respirator

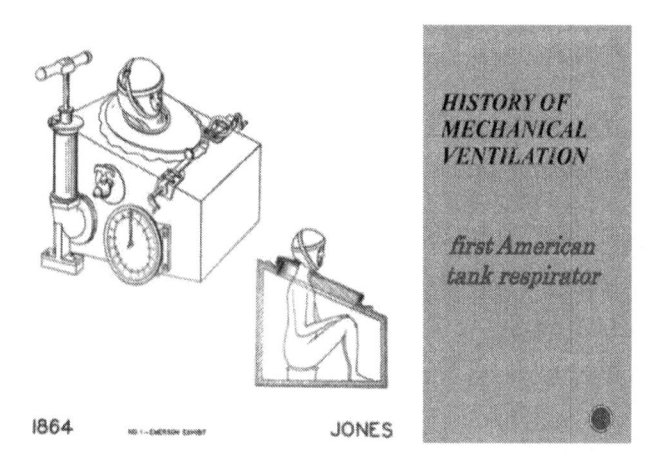

1864   JONES

This was an arduous task, requiring strength and concentration, just even to get each patient into the chair, notwithstanding the monotony of working the pump. So, I devised a rota, on an hourly basis – a nurse to be in control of each machine for an hour at a time.

There had been a couple of young lads, who had turned up for the interviews. I picked out two, both about 14 years of age, Kevin Barker and Jimmy Jackson. I explained to them that they were needed to lift patients to the respirator and move beds, as required. I wasn't sure if they would be strong enough to do this task – they looked quite weak and undernourished and their clothes were ragged.

"Ah, way's strang. Way con left onything. Way mayt looek pueny but way just nayds fayding up a moight. Way've 'ad nothing much in ways of deenners, but way con di it. Just gee us a tray. Way're men neow. Way's bin warking sin way was 10."

"Ok. I'll sit on this seat and I want you to pick me up, with one of you either side, with one hand under the chair and one hand supporting the back of the chair, and move me, without toppling me over, to the other side of the room. Can you do that?"

They certainly had a go. There was a bit of a wobble at first but they got me safely to the other side of the room.

"Ok, that was fine. You will also be required to do the washing of bedding and nightwear, towels and so on, Oh, also help in the kitchen. There's water laid on here, so no fetching of buckets of water from whatever local stream is nearby."

"Or, but thut's wemen's wark. Way wonna di wemen's wark. Thet's not fer the loiks of us."

"It may have been considered to be women's work, but that is only because men didn't want to do the work. It is in fact a very strenuous, back-breaking task, that no women should be doing. It will definitely built up your muscles and I can see from your arms that you haven't got much muscle definition. Take it or leave it."

I went on, "Did you know that the best cooks are, according to the French, men. In France they call them 'chefs'."

Kevin replied, "Or, olraight. Is theer a foncy Frinch neeme fer min doing the wushing an'o?"

So, just to give them something to fit the bill, I said. "Now, let's see. Yes, you can be 'lingeurs' (pronounced 'langure'). So, are we up for the job?

They both looked pleased as Punch at this name and turned out to be good workers, in their new brown coats. Of course, getting good, nourishing meals, they soon filled out and became strong lads.

So, the ward was up and running and being kept clean and medicine, and clinical apparatus, as it was at the time, being provided.

Remembering forward in time, yes, we had an array of medical facilities, equipment and medicine, with trained nurses and doctors doing the best for patients, with new innovations being discovered regularly in treatment for various diseases. But, there was a downside. Nurses were highly trained, yes, but cleanliness of the wards, which in the later 19th century had been undertaken by the nurses and overseen by the Matron, had now gone out to contract workers. You'd think, fine, OK, the wards are being kept clean, but there had been an influx of biological germs that these contract workers were not able to get rid of just by peripheral cleaning, as carried out by the contract workers, such as MRSA. People were entering wards with, for example a broken bone, catching this germ and dying. Elderly people were objecting to being sent to hospital, in the fear that they would never come out again. This was a great worry to them. So, following Florence Nightingale having set up schools to train nurses, and ensuring part of their job was cleaning, the wards in the late 19th century were actually cleaner. That doesn't say much for progress.

CHAPTER 15 – THE WORKHOUSE INFIRMARY

"I hope I'm not boring you, John. It's just that there's so much to catch up on over the years."

"Thut's alreet, Jane. Eet's no as ef ah'm goin' onyweer fest. No, ah'd loik te 'ere whut yer've bin doein'. Yer've difinitely no bin settin' on yer becksaide allov thay'se yayrs."

"Quite true, but nor have you, my dear. Anyway, we'll have something to eat and then I'll continue where I left off."

Whilst I was preparing the meal I asked John how he was feeling and if, maybe he was up for a short walk.

"Oh, ah'm olraight. Ah'm in nowe payne. Yer, mebbee ah cod di wi' a beet o' ixercayse – nowe 'ills but. Ah donna eef ah'm up fer 'ills."

"That's good. How about a slow walk to the Red Cow? You could have a beer or two sitting in the sunshine at the back, looking over the farms and fields? Take a jacket though, just in case it gets a bit windy."

"Thut sarnds gooed. Eet'll git may owt've thayse fur wolls en ah cod di wi' a paint."

So, after lunch, we took a slow walk to the Red Cow. There was a little bit of an incline to get to it, but I could see that John wasn't going to miss out on his pint.

The view south, sloping down towards Caverswall was spectacular, just a patchwork of farms. Of course, we could have gone to the Windmill, but there's a better view from the Red Cow and we'd be away from the dust and smell from the horse and carts travelling along the main Ash Bank Road.

The Red Cow was a small pub. It didn't have the extension at the back for the restaurant. That was built in the 20th century. All the farmers got in there with their dogs. It was a bit rough and smokey, with a coal fire blazing in the winter, and had low beams but seats were provided at the back for anyone wanting to sit there.

So, over our pints, I continued with my story.

The ward was up and running so I took the opportunity to look around at the other wards. I hadn't realised that a workhouse was part of the complex. There was a set of rules pinned to a wall, stating that anyone 'desiring' to enter a workhouse as an inmate (not casual) having received his (or her) proper form of admission, is taken first of all to the new receiving ward.

"I mean, John, did anyone 'desire' to enter a workhouse! They would have been at the end of their tether, starving, ill, dying even, to be driven to enter a workhouse."

"Anyway, the notice continued that their clothes were to be taken away, thoroughly disinfected, and stowed away in case they may be required again. Then he or she is taken to a warm bathroom to be given a hot bath, after which a night-gown is supplied and the applicant is shown to a room accommodating twelve good beds. First thing in the morning the applicant would be examined by the doctor, and on that gentleman's certificate, is placed in whatever department he (or she) is fitted for. He is now on probation, and at the next following meeting of the Guardians his case is gone into; and if found deserving, he is allowed to stay in the house; if not, the alternative course is taken."

"Thut ol sarnds very naice, naice worem bath en a gooed bid, wi a doctor te looek efter yer."

"Yes, but don't you believe it. What I found would make you turn in your boots and run."

My story:
The reality was that, to receive medical attention under the poor law, a person first had to be declared a pauper and it was never envisaged that paupers should receive medical attention. The New Poor Law was designed to deter paupers and not to offer them free hospital treatment or specialised care in institutions. The Commissioners had no long-term plan for larger institutions and therefore reluctant to accept the fact that many workhouses were being increasingly viewed as hospitals. From what I could ascertain, I would consider three quarters of the inmates were ill with some sort of disease or other. The new Poor Law poured scorn and brutality on both general practitioners and pauper patients.

Joseph Rogers had helped form the Poor Law medical Officer's Association in 1867, in London, an important pressure group working for further reform of poor law medical services, but, obviously these reforms had not reached Stoke.

As I made my way around, I heard a woman moaning. I managed to speak to her. She seemed so weak and her voice was hoarse, making it difficult to hear her, but I managed to ascertain that she had recently given birth. The baby had been taken away from her and she had no way of finding out where it was or even if it was a girl or boy – no-one had told her. They'd put her on a starvation diet for the past nine days, just a bowl of stinking gruel a day, that had bits floating in it that could have been flies or maggots.

"Thah gee'ing may nowt proper te ate 'cos ah'm not marrit, thee telt may", she managed to whisper. I said I'd bring her something to eat but I'd have to sneak it in as I could see people watching me.

Wandering around were a number of what I would call "lost souls" shouting out abuse and interfering with patients in their beds. They looked dirty and ill-kempt, some having torn out their hair and torn and dirtied their clothes. So, these people, obviously suffering with mental distress and illness, were allowed to walk around, unguarded amongst obviously physically ill people, and to abuse them in any way they wanted to. Obviously they didn't know what they were doing but, there was no-one to prevent them doing so.

The infirmary had it own bakery, laundry and workshops. Out in the open I saw a group of men noisily beating at carpets. Most were coughing and spluttering from the dust that was rising up out of the carpets. On questioning one of the men, I found out that this was one of the tasks set him. I asked him how long he'd had the cough and he said that he came in with it.

"Ah wus dine on may uppers – codna wark. May chist 'urts whin ah cughs en ah cughs up blod somtarms. Thee puts may on thus wark – macks may cugh woss. Ah conna see onythin' utherwayse ah gits a baytin' missel."

This man was obviously ill but still made to do heavy manual work in dusty conditions. He continued that he would be got up out of bed at 5.45 in the morning and be working until 8pm. Meals were adequate but very stodgy and no talking was allowed during meal times. He had come in with his wife and two children and he had been separated from them – he'd just see his wife occasionally through a gap in the wall. His children had been sent to an orphanage.

On going back inside I realised that there were in fact no nurses or doctors that I could see. The infirmary seemed to be run by the patients. I actually saw someone washing his hands and face in the water from his bedchamber pot. In fact there was no water tap that I could see and, going into the syphilis ward, which had eight inmates, there was just an old towel, for the use of all of these eight patients and which looked like it had been there all week – just a soaking, dirty, bedraggled, germ-filled rag.

"Since then, John, money had been allocated to Stoke and Wolstanton for building of one hundred and fifty-five workhouse infirmaries. I kept excerpts from the newspapers of building work that has happened over the years and brought these out with me."

Reading through these extracts I told John that Stoke has taken advantage of this expansion but Woltanton has only expanded once. An old school was turned into wards to provide additional accommodation for forty patients and there's talk of providing a small infectious hospital, probably with three or four beds for either sex in the next couple of years, taking into account the number of beds required.

I carried on, "In 1874, a new infectious hospital was operating, but was described by Inspector Dansey as 'only adequate'. Later that same year, as a consequence of another outbreak of smallpox, a further purpose-built wooden structure was erected at a cost of £303.15s, to accommodate an additional eighty-nine sick patients. Even today, John, after all this building work, there's still a shortage of accommodation. Some workhouse infirmaries are even refusing to take infectious cases on the basis that the chance of recovery is less than for those who remain in their homes. Plus, in the old infirmary there has been a report that patients are being put five in a bed in the general sick wards. I'll just read out the description of conditions, if that's alright with you?"

John nodded, so I read out to him, "The additions to the old infirmary are most un-satisfactory as there is poor ventilation throughout. The bath is in the cellar; the stairs are dangerously steep and the lavatory arrangements defective. It is ill-adapted to have an additional storey."

"Sa, Jane, eet looeks loik things 've got woss sin yer was warking theer in '71."

"Yes, these buildings just were not made to accommodate so many people coming to live in the six towns."

My story continued:
I'd looked around for nursing staff while I was on this visit. As I said, I felt I was being watched, not just watched, I was being followed by patients who obviously had mental health issues. I didn't feel safe but turned towards them, told them I was Nurse Knight and ordered them back to their beds. They went, thank goodness. I suppose they were just being curious. Anyway, I didn't find any nurses or doctors in the wards I visited. The patients seemed to be fending for themselves. I did manage to find one patient, Susan Collins, who seemed to be 'in charge' of the other patients. I started talking to her and managed to glean that she was in fact an inmate of the workhouse, but thought well enough to work in the infirmary. She hadn't had any nursing training, but it seemed she had been given the job of looking after the ward when Nurse Abott wasn't there. Nurse Abott had gone off shift now. Susan went on to say that Nurse Abott had no particular nursing qualifications and no special knowledge or aptitude for the job. She was there more in line of a domestic servant – providing basic care of patients and cleaning and washing.

When I next got back home, John, I looked up anything I could find relating to workhouse infirmaries. I've got it here. I'll read it to you. There was a General Consolidated Order of 1847 that sets out the duties of workhouse nurses." I started to read, 'The duties of workhouse nurses is simply to attend the sick, to administer to them all medicines and medical applications, according to the direction of the medical officer; to inform the medical officer of any defects observed in the arangements in sick lying-in wards; and to take care that a light was kept at night in the sick wards. The workhouse nurses are required to be sober and capable of reading and understanding the medical officer's instructions.

I got talking to a gentleman on the ward, a Mr Lambert. He was an educated man but had obviously fallen on hard times. He was desperate to get out and was busy writing a letter to the governors. He told me his story."

'I entered Stoke workhouse and was seen by the Master and he placed me into the Idiot Ward. Here one of the idiots was carried in bleeding from the nose. The idiots kept yelling, shouting out. I was in no fit state to see what all the shouting was about – my chest hurt. I asked someone why I was on the Idiot Ward, I mean, I'm no idiot. He said it was common for the nurse to place sick patients in the Idiot Ward. There is no partition to keep the idiots from rambling into any of the wards.

Mr Ashfort, the assistant or medical officer, visited the next day. I tried to call out that I was having chest pains, but he left without seeing me. He came again and again, without seeing me. I told the nurse I needed to see the doctor but she just turned to me and said something I shan't repeat. I asked to see the Master but she refused.

On Thursday I was taken off the Idiot Ward and placed in the old men's sick ward then seen by Mr Garner, the medical officer. I told him my chest was painful, on the right hand side,' Indicating where it hurt. "I know", he said, "now shut up" was his reply. 'After sounding me, he pointed to the nurse, "This man wants little or no medicine, just give him the opening mixture." The nurse then presented me with a large cup full of dark mixture, I found out later that this medicine is more suitable for horses than sickly humans and had been nicknamed "Black Jack" by the patients.

This place is nothing more than a cesspit. I want out. Get me out, please. I'm writing a letter to the Governors but I don't know what good that will do. You're just visiting. You won't have seen much but, just open your eyes. You wouldn't believe what I've seen since I've been here. Every day I see patients comb their heads in pursuit of finding lice in large numbers. There are no facilities for personal cleanliness – can you see any basins Nurse Knight? No, there aren't any. Patients are washing themselves in chamber pots, others don't bother washing as they feel repugnance to wash in a chamber pot not used by themselves. There are no towels, no soap and but three chamber pots for seven men. I have seen the old men's ward, which was my day ward, where for three days successively, it was without soap of any kind, hard or soft. There were here but two small towels for 11 or12 men. I have myself washing these several times when they were shamefully filthy and could procure no soap for the purpose. I had to go to the laundry in the basement to find water and me feeling really crook, but I forced myself to do it.'

He was right, the whole place was a stinking mess. I left Mr Lambert and took a tour of the old men's ward. I saw two beds in it with very filthy covering. In one bed a man and in the other four boys, two at each end. I spoke to the inmate nurse, "Do all the boys have diarrhoea?" Not looking at the boys, she replied, "Thah ol but free of eet – eet mun bay sommit thah've ate or filth or a beet o' the two."

I returned to Mr Lambert, "All I get to eat is bread, butter and coffee for breakfast and again in the evening, The coffee or tea is all but cold, the bread is half-cooked and the butter is rancid. I've seen patients scrape off the butter. For dinner they serve us rice and broth, although the rice is musty and old and tastes like it's been baked or boiled in some watery matter, certainly not all milk. The broth has no vegetables and any meat is too tough to chew.

There are no knives or forks or spoons. You've got to eat with your fingers or sup the broth, unless you can borrow cutlery from the others.'

I went to ask the nurse about this lack of cutlery and got the reply, "Oh, theer allowed but theer not supplied. Ef theer's knoives en sich or medicines eet's 'cos I gees 'em ite. Ah *'as te* bay 'em iyta may ourn paye en ah gits just £20 the yayre, so thee gits whut thee gits."

"Sa, th'enfarmary wus in a raight stayte. God 'elp 'em."

"It gets worse, John.

I found a locked room and thought it must be for cleaning utensils. "What's in this room Susan?"

"Oh, yer mussna go in theer."

"Whatever for? I'm looking for soap for the ward."

"Theer's somwon coms in ivery sa eften te say te the peeshients in theer. Say, theer've go' the pox. Shay's anuther enmeete loik may, but shay's 'ad the pox hersen, sa the Master 'as go' 'er en to trayt 'em."

"Do you mean to say there's a patient in there – in a walk-in cupboard room?"
"Yes, miss."

"Well, I need to see what's going on. It's alright. I have had a smallpox inoculation, so I'm immune. Please open the door."

"Eef yer insist, miss." and she duly opened the door for me.
What greated me at first was a stench of faeces. It was dark so I asked for a candle. On looking further I saw the eyes staring at me out of the gloom. I called out, "How many of you

211

are here?" The weak, distressed answer came from a young boy, no older than eight, shielding his eyes from the light from the doorway. "Six Mrs."

"When did the doctor last come to see you?"

"Ah dunno, Mrs. Theer's a woman coms every so often to feed us and clean us and I've seen the door open, with a man looking in, but that's all, en way 'anna sayn the woman fer som tarm. Way're 'starved deeth. Ah dunno if Peter 'ere is aloive. Ah canna seem te wake 'im."

I stepped over bodies lying on a soiled mattress and checked all of the children. One of the boys had indeed died. I got Susan to go fetch the other woman. At last she arrived. She was aged and quite infirm herself and I could smell she'd been drinking. However, between the two of us, we managed to wrap poor Peter in a sheet and take him to the mortuary.

I then commenced to berate Susan. "This is a dreadful state of affairs. I've never seen anything like it. Clean up the room and the boys and feed them. I will be advising the Master of the appaling situation I have found these poor boys in. I find this workhouse infirmary to be unfit for human habitation and you and the rest of the so-called staff here, are for the high jump." She just shrugged her shoulders. "OK. By your reaction, I can see that means nothing to you. Well, obviously you're drunk and I can only summise that you get the alcohol in exchange for doing this work. As you have not carried out your tasks, *you will no longer get access to alcohol. "Ah but ah nayds it, miss. Dosna tack may drenk awee fram may."*

"Ah, so I'm hitting home now, am I. Well, I'm afraid it's too late to bemoan your fate – drink and any other privileges will be taken away from you, now get on with cleaning up. I'll be watching you."

As for no attention from a doctor, that was something else. I'd have to approach the Master and also take this further, with Dr Knight's assistance.

I went to see Dr Knight afterwards and told him what I had discovered.

"Yes, hmmm. I know a Royal Commission was set up in 1869 to investigate serious public health issues. I shall take this matter to them. From what I understand though, no money has been allocated for medication to doctors at workhouses. There is no provision for drugs so that the doctor has to pay out of his own stipend for any he prescribes, so they just turn a blind eye. Also, this said, there's no money for allocation of trained nurses. As you have found out on your visit, there is just enough money for a single paid nurse to oversee thirty or forty patients, and this means that everything done for the sick is by inmates. They have nothing to gain if they do the duty assigned and nothing to lose if they do it badly. The fact that being deemed able-bodied women, they are still workhouse inmates, who have been proved, prima facie, not to be of high character; so most of them are not disposed to take much

trouble in attending to helpless folk requiring assistance, in various respects, by night or day. Pauper nurses simply receive extra privileges in the form of food, alcohol or token cash payments for their special duties, such as a glass of gin for laying-out the dead and other repulsive duties. At Stoke, the guardians have set to work children under the age of thirteen to perform nursing and domestic duties."

"Yes, I've seen all of this first hand. But there is money, they've built the hospital here and extended it - the guardians just have to be influenced or persuaded to overcome their reluctance to pay for services, plus institutions need to be set up for the training of nurses."

"Your Florence Nightingale you are so fond of quoting, has indeed set up a training scheme at the workhouse infirmary in Liverpool, and this has been running since 1865. It has been financed by a local benefactor, William Rathbone, so yes, a delegate must approach the benefactors in this area to do the same. I will see what can be done."

So, John, that Royal Commission became the Local Government Board in 1871, with responsibilities for public health as well as the poor law. Changes were made. In most workhouses nursing was to be supervised by a Matron, usually a role taken on by the Master's wife.

In 1875 guardians at Stoke appointed a properly 'qualified nurse for the male side of the workhouse, where previously, as I have said, the duties had been carried out by pauper inmates, The position was advertised at £15 per annum but, unfortunately received no applications. The LGB agreed that the guardians could increase this to £19 or even £25 to secure the right appointment. During this time, however, pauper inmates were still being used in the hospital. The medical officer finally agreed it was necessary to appoint a trained night nurse to replace the pauper inmate who would sit up all night, plus they'd, at last, come to realise that inmate nurses could not be relied upon.

Getting qualified staff seemed to be a hit and run way of working. No-one wanted to take the responsibility and they blamed each other if the candidate appeared not to be up to the job. From what I understand, appointments were first made by the guardians and then these were submitted to the LGB for final approval. Sometimes references were followed up, sometimes not. So-called qualified nurses, were proved after their appointment, to be none the such and one appointment was made where it was found the candidate was illiterate, and she was still offered the position.

In one case, the medical officer complained to the guardians, saying he had not been represented on the appointments panel, or involved in the selection process, so objected to the person appointed. It was just chaotic. Not here, but in Leicester, I heard that two nurses had been appointed, one had previously been a machinist and the other in domestic service – and this, despite pressure by the LGB that only trained nurses should be appointed."

"Poppycock. 'Ow deed thee raych theer positions. Saymes loik thee codna organase a pess-up in a breuwery." replied John, "One sade dinna knar whut t'uther sade wus doing, wi' the guerdians appiynting 'oo thee wunted, na carring abite suitability or expairience, plus the LGB war ixpected t'approoeve sich appiyntments wi'ite quistion!"

"That's it to a tee, John."

So, even today, they've not got a qualified nursing force. I hear all sorts of happenings, one where a nurse left her patients overnight to visit another part of the workhouse. She's been asked to resign – and another case where a nurse has been asked to resign over her ill-treatment of an inmate. It seems she placed a 74-year-old female patient into a bath of cold water as a form of punishment."

"Thah no o bed thoogh, shorely? Theer's gotta bay som gooeduns?

"Quite true, and these have been given credit for their work. Plus staffing levels have increased to five nurses in the sick ward and two with the imbeciles and, low and behold, the medical officer actually attends daily."

"Doss 'e just attend or is 'e medickeeting the peeshients?"

"I can see you've been listening, John. Very good, that's the cynical part of your mind coming through. And too true. Who knows? I hope so, that's all I can say. We can only hope someone is overseeing him and the nurses.

Anyway, John, I think we should be making our way back now."

CHAPTER 15 – SPECTRES

John was tired and went for a lie down. It may have been the couple of beers, it may have been the exercise but, obviously, he still wasn't well, although he was getting there and, given a bit of time, he would be fine. It was good to have these days with him and I was beginning to feel whole again, after so many years on my own - just having someone to talk to. There was still, however, a distance between us and I couldn't see how that would ever be healed. He was still wary of me and what he saw as my past indiscretions and, obviously, the murder of Geoffrey, no matter how indirect, which he could never forgive me for. But, oh how I longed for him just to put his arm around me. It would never happen though what with his heart-felt beliefs that I was a witch of some kind. He just couldn't trust me any more and there was nothing I could do to win over his trust again. I knew deep in my heart that he still had some kind of love for me and he would love to hold me close, but that his fears and mistrust, just blocked any movement towards me. I was afraid to make any move towards him, even hold his hand, as I knew he would just back away, and that would be that.

That awful hallucination came to mind again, the inky blackness of the water and the relief at seeing his hand close by. So close but still such a gap between us.

Then my thoughts strayed to the phenomenon I saw in Bridle Path, the ghost of myself from the future. She came to warn me of the danger Alfred was in. Was she watching over me? Did she know all that I was doing? Oh if only I could summon her up when needed, to help me. I needed her now to get through to John – to tell him the truth. It was no good praying, she was not God, I didn't even know if she were an angel, she certainly didn't have wings. Maybe she was another hallucination. Oh, it was just too much. What were these apparitions?

My mind went to Elizabeth Meigh telling me that she had seen Job Meigh after he had died. His ghostly form was at the top of the winding stairs, mouthing the word "sorry" over and over again. I'd heard so many stories from people of ghostly figures being seen, figures who had died violent premature deaths or were not 'at rest' for some reason on other, or figures just appearing where they used to walk, so I wasn't the only person to see such figures. Why could only some people see these images? Yes, I suppose there were 'sensitives' - people who were attuned to the wave-length of these ghostly figures and could channel their thoughts, but why weren't all people, who were still tied to this earthly life for some reason or other, appearing as ghostly figures – there would be billions through the ages – think of all the wars that had happened and murders. Why weren't these people haunting where they died or used to live? I didn't understand this. The church, especially the Catholic church, had their own means of dispelling these earth-bound ghostly figures – an exorcism - sending them on their way, but I wasn't religious and I didn't want to send my future ghostly self away. If she was here to protect and warn me, I still needed her.

There was another story Elizabeth Meigh had told me. I really didn't understand it. It was a warning, but not to me directly. It was some years after Geoffrey had been killed and after the death of Job Meigh.

"My maid came in to the room as I was sitting by the fire reading."

"Excuse me m'am," she said, curtseying, "beg pardon for disturbing you, but I've been hearing strange noises coming from the nursery, you know, the old classroom. Well, it fare well bothers me and I'm right frittened. I've also seen weird lights, green and horange lights coming from the room a couple of times. I told Dinah about it and we both got our courage up to peak round the door ….. well I don't want to be a fusser but I'm right flummoxed and allova flusker."

"Go on girl."

"Well, Dinah telt me to come tell you… but, well, and I'm all a dither, after what we've seen."

"She could see me getting a bit ill tempered waiting for her to spit it out what she and Dinah had seen, so she finally managed to get out….."

".. Well, the room was fair freeze haskers. I could see own my breathe. We looks round the door and there was this light, sort of shimmering horange and green. We couldn't make it out at first, *but then it took a sort of shape – that of a young lad.... I think, ma'm, we've sin a boggert."*

"Well, Jane, I can admit I was taken aback by the thought that we had a ghost, but I got up and made my way to the old schoolroom. I wanted to see whatever it was, for myself. I looked hesitantly around the door and, sure enough, saw the orange and green shimmering light for myself. I cautiously entered the room and tentatively spoke to light, saying who I was. You'd never believe it but I heard a voice coming from the light, the voice of a young boy. It said, 'M'am, I have to warn you.... There is a servant intending to betray a secret – a secret about your friend, Jane Wood that you have inwardly suspected is true, but couldn't quite believe, and have thus said nothing. I asure you that your innermost beliefs are real, no matter how strange. However, this servant intends to tell this secret to all who will listen and, in doing so, will bring downfall on you for befriending the lady. The servant's name is Tom Forrester."

"Well, Jane, I needn't tell you I was completely taken aback. Not least that my suspicions about you were true."

"So, you know my secret." I replied.

"I do. It all makes sense now, no matter how bizarre. It explains how you know things that no-one else could possibly know. Job, being Job, never put two and two together and called you a witch *or deranged. He would have had you whipped if he could, but I didn't want to lose our friendship as you'd been such a great help to me especially with your devised exercises for me, following my brain haemorrhage – training that no-one else in the world had established. You got me on my feet again, quite litterally and saved me from a wretched bed-ridden life – Job not withstanding, that is!*

"Please do not tell my secret, it would be my undoing." Tom Forrester was the one I had taught at school, and who I believed had something to do with the murder of my Geoffrey.

"I wouldn't dream of it, my girl. According to the spirit, it would be my own undoing too. You will wish to know that, what I did next, was to request Tom Forrester come to see me. I told him that I knew he was about to betray a family secret and that this amounted to no less than treachery. However, the young scallywag denied knowing anything, and yes, I had no proof, but it was a warning, that I hoped would frighten him into submission.

However, that wasn't the end of it, Jane. I was out riding with Tom Forrester, acting as escort, riding slowly back via Bridle Path. You know, that part where the path is dark and overgrown with overhead tree branches linking above from both sides of the path and cutting out the sunlight.

All of a sudden an apparition appeared in front of us. I believe the horses could see the apparition too as they whinnied and stamped, reversed a bit, even tried to bolt, but we managed, somehow, to hold them in check.

The apparition spoke, "Tom."

Tom was aghast, "You know my name?"

The apparition spoke again, a youthful voice eerily, fading in and out, "I know you Tom, and I know what you are about to make known about Jane Wood..... DO NOT! .... If you do, there will be dire consequences."

"Why, what ....will happen? Who are you.....who were you? What ...are you going to do ...to me?" Tom's voice was naturally shaky.
"You know me Tom, and you know what you did."

There seemed to be a look of recognition come over Tom, who had dismounted. He stepped back, seeming to want to run away.

"You've got nowhere to run to Tom." The spectre shouted. "If you repeat what you think you know, I will haunt you for the rest of your life. What you are about to say is untrue. You do not have the facts. If you continue I will guarantee the rest of your life will not be worth living. I will make sure your family perishes, you will not be able to find work and you will die in torment and starvation."

Tom was still shaking, but had gathered his wits about him to some extent. He started to speak, hesitantly at first, stuttering. "What.. 've I.... to be afeared... of you." Then he gained more confidence and stood up straight. "You're just little. You can't do much to me. I've grown big since last time I saw you. And what are these facts. I've no idea what you mean."

There was a sudden woosh of moving mist and the frantic braying of an invisible horse then, gradually, out of the mist, another apparition slowly took shape, a man astride a rampant horse, wildly pawing its front hooves through the mist. The rider was violently thrashing, with his whip, through the vapourous air before him.

I almost fainted, I could tell you, but I had to use all my wits to check my horse to prevent it about-turning and running and throwing me to the ground. I held on tightly to my horse's neck, to stop myself falling. Tom's horse had already galloped off in fright, but I had to stay. I needed to find out what this spectre had to say. Was he a ghost of things that had been or a warning of things that were to come.

The rider finally controlled the horse and brought it to stand alongside the other spectre. I recognised him immediately – it was Job – mounted majestically on his black stallion. My heart was leaping with fear and trepidation as to what this spectre of my husband wanted.

An eerie, echoing voice addressed Tom.

"The facts are not for you to know or understand. Keep your sordid tales to yourself for the rest of your life. Do not ever disrespect the good name of Mrs Wood or allow any other person to do so, for fear of your own life. This secret must remain her secret. Do you understand the consequences, Tom? I know now your part in what happened to young Geoffrey Wood on that fateful night, and I will not keep this secret if you betray Mrs Wood. I will be watching you."

By this time Tom had fallen to his knees he was so frightened. He was crying now, almost prostrate on the ground. Please, please go away, leave me be."

"Swear, Tom, swear on your life, you miserable piece of humanity."

I swear,…. I swear I will not tell a living soul, as what I thought I knew, is untrue. ….. I will not bear false witness,…. in the name of God the Father, the Son and the Holy Ghost, so help me God."

At that, Tom attempted to look up and saw the spectres fade away.

……

Mrs Meigh continued, "It was such a frightening spectre that I don't think Tom was ever himself afterwards. He never said what the secret was all about and I've never heard any rumours about you, not even from Job after he sacked you – he wouldn't tell me anything anyway, as you know we do not speak to each other apart from common courtesies, of which these are few and far between. It's all very intriguing, and I know what I know, but I don't know how it came about. All I know is that I mustn't enquire. I must say, though, that I have every faith in you. Rumours are rumours and easily spread when there is no foundation in them. I do not listen to gossip. What I will tell you though, Jane, is that the first spectre, even though menacing, seemed to be that of a young boy, not unlike your own Geoffrey."

I was astounded. Could Geoffrey still be protecting me and keeping my secret from beyond the grave? My sweet Geoffrey.

CHAPTER 16 – ST MARY'S CHURCH

Thinking about young Tom, swearing his oath of silence in the name of God the Father, the Son and the Holy Ghost, reminded me of when St Mary's Church was built in Bucknall. The corner stone was laid on Wednesday, 19th April 1854 and was reported in the Staffordshire Advertiser the following Saturday, April 22nd. John and I were no longer together. The next morning, I reminded John of this great event.

"Everyone was there and anyone who was anyone. I happened to meet up with you there, in the crowd. I don't know how happy you were to see me, but you didn't move off."

"Yer, eet was thrutched, ah codna go anywhere, so ah 'ad to put up wi' yer."

"Oh, that's nice. Nothing like a bit of friendly chat for old time's sake."

"Well, ah codna say yer bayin' pushed en shoved int cride. So, ah steeyed.

"Always protecting me, ay John, whatever I do."

"Ef yer say so, en ah thowght ah wus seef - yer codna put a spill on may on chorch gruns."

"Oh, John, you're unrelenting!"

John laughed at that and gave me a little squeeze of my arm. I was so taken aback I tweaked his nose, then he pushed me away again. Nevertheless, he was still smiling. It was so good to see him smile in my presence again. Maybe the ice was finally beginning to crack and I wanted to keep hold of that little slither of tenderness.

"Yes, I'm completely powerless on church ground, every witch knows that." I continued in the same way, giving him a cheeky smile.

I left it at that and carried on about the church. "Yes, the old church was nothing but a ruin. It had stood there for, I don't know, years and years anyway, but had got so dilapidated that it was beyond restoration and, besides that, it was quite inadequate to serve the number of people coming into the neighbourhood."

"Yer, payple wunted sommit beegger en mer ilegant en a conseederable amiynt o monney wus obteened fram Lichfield Diocesan Chorch Society en Incorporated Society, as will as parish reetes end praivate subscreeptions."

"I believe the ground to be used for the new church was adjacent to the old church and was given over by R Sneyd Esq of Keele Hall."

"Int' mayntarm wark comminced on dimoleshing th'old belding. As yer sayd, th'old chorch wus encient. Ah belayve thee trayed te rebuild eet in 1716 fram staynes tacken fram 'Ulton Abbey. The chancel erch en chancel etsel war browght o'er, fram th'abbey, olthowgh at deefferent tarms."

"Yes, it was quaint and picturesque but not remarkable for any beauty of form or detail, and was surrounded by groups of fine old yew trees. I would think it was originally a small chapelry attached to Hutton Abbey up to the period of the dissolution of the monasteries by Henry VIII.

"The neuw chorch wus te bay built abite fifty yerds to the sithe o' the ol one, on a beet 'igher grun en bay an attrective addetion te vellage ginerally, wi' the spayre bayin' a strayking criwn te th'ole idifice. Ah monaged te 've a looek at the plans afore'and. Thee wanted a nave abite 60ft lung, wi a sithe ailse abite sem lingth."

"Hold on there, John. You know I like to keep snippets from the newspapers. I think I've got something in my box about the church from the Staffordshire Advertiser. Let me see....... Yes, here it is. You're right. I'll read it: 'It will be built in the early English style, and will consist of a nave, 63 feet long by 21 ft wide; a south aisle the same length, by 10 feet 9 inches wide; a south or children's aisle, 27 feet 6 inches long by 14 feet wide; and a small chancel aisle and vestry. A porch will ornament the south side, and the steeple on the north side will form another porch entrance for adults and children. It will accommodate upwards of 500 persons, and will be heated by an apparatus, for which a vault is provided beneath. The whole will be built of stone from the Werrington quarries. The interior of the roofs and the seats will be frames open of deal, and stained and varnished; and the roofs outside will be covered with tiles. The base of the steeple only will, for the present, be carried up. Messrs. Ward and Son, of Hanley, are the architects, and the contractor Mr Thos. Reeves of Werrington. The estimated total cost of the building, when completed is £2,300; but the present contract will not be more than £1,850.'

As you said, there was a host of people, some estimated about a thousand turned up with plenty of very important people with several elegantly dressed ladies. Smith Child, the MP was there to lay the cornerstone. Job Meigh was there too and his son, William, all with their wives, a couple of Reverends, including Mr H Sneyd of Wetley Rocks and church wardens. From what I remember, these dignatories were at the head of a procession, followed by school children, the church choir, architects, builder and workmen. The choir and children were singing a hymn, they were sweet and angelic-looking, in their white choir smocks, didn't you think so, John?" John just nodded.

"Then the service commenced with a reading by the rector. After the reading, the stone was laid by Sir Smith Child, who then gave a very long and drawn-out religious speech. "

"Yer, ah rimember eet baying a beet wendy, but lockily eet dinna reen. Way was stondin' theer fer eejes, lestning to 'im. E's a gradeley mon, but a lung wendsoc,thut 'e is."

"Now, now, John. You should respect your elders and betters. Anyway, I know him. I met him at a party Job Meigh held at Ash

Hall the year of the riots . He was also at the various magistrate meetings held about the riots, two of which I attended. He did well for himself, marrying Sarah, an heiress, daughter of Richard Clarke Hill of Stallington Hall, Stone. Then became a Conservative MP. He's a good man, a philanthropist, contributing annually to the Staffordshire Infirmary as well as many other good causes, such as supporting medical institutions in Tunstall and has done a lot of work to develop Tunstall. He actually foresaw the riots, owing to the lack of food and work and the termination of poor relief and was trying to get something done."

"True, ah soppose, en it wus a gooed, religious spaych, sooetable fer th'evint en ivveraone wus leestening intintly."

"Anyway, the whole speech has been recorded in the paper. I've no idea how they took it all down word for word. The reporter must have taken a Pitman's course. I couldn't see Job Meigh balling him out for taking shorthand, as he did me but, then again, this was 12 years on and times change. Do you think you could bear me to read the speech?"

"Olraight, com on, effin yer mun, ah knahs yer daying te."

"Ok, here goes, I'll take a deep breath:

'Mr Smith Child afterwards ascended the stone, and eloquently addressed the assembly. He observed that they had met together that day upon a most important occasion, to lay the corner stone of an edifice, which would hereafter be dedicated to the most important uses – the uses of the utmost and deepest moment to every child of man. To most important uses, inasmuch as they might well trust that within those walls would be enunciated, those principles, on the holding fast of which man's temporal and spiritual happiness   depended – and depended in so far that they were coincident with and could only be secured by his obeying the precepts of the Gospel. Without the sunshine of the Holy Spirit being within him, he must fall into misery and debasement, and that sunshine could only exist where there was a regenerated heart and an anxious desire, under the blessing and assistance of God, to obey the everlasting precepts He had laid down for the guidance and direction of mankind.

He could not but feel flattered in having been selected by them to perform that interesting ceremony, inasmuch as he had no connection by property or residence with the parish in which they were assembled. He could only attribute the selection to the public position he had the honour to fill. As holding that position there might perhaps be some degree of fitness in deputing him to fulfil the duty he had just performed, for that position must ever remind him of an obligation, as he maintained it was, incumbent upon him as the representative of a great constituency such as that, namely, to uphold the great landmarks of our country, amongst the most important of which were those attached to the fabric of the Church. He believed that the Reformed Apostolic Church, to which he trusted the majority of those he was addressing, belonged, was, under God, one great means of maintaining the welfare of promoting the prosperity, and consolidating the strength of this great nation; in as much as its strength depended not so much upon externals as upon the inherent spirit of its people. Our Church was the great bulwark of the Reformation; it was at once a bulwark against Popery on the one hand, and against infidelity on the other. It had been the practice of mankind in all ages to erect buildings for every public purpose, and they lavished their wealth in adorning and rendering magnificent such edifices. They erected monuments to commemorate **noble deeds,** halls of justice, and temples dedicated to the cultivation of the arts and literature, and also rejoiced to adorn, and render worthy of habitation, the royal palaces of sovereigns, but the building, whose walls were now beginning to rise around them, combined all those qualifications. Would it not be a monument to commemorate the greatest deeds, which had affected the welfare of the human race? It would surely commemorate the creation of the world, the creation and the fall of man, and more than that, the greatest blessings conferred on man, his redemption through the Son of God. It would surely, then, be dedicated to great and noble uses. The history of man from the earliest and most remote ages would be there, declared for the guidance and consolation of future generations. Would not strains of poetry be heard within those walls, strains which had passed from lips touched by the Divine fire of inspiration, from the sublime Psalmist of Israel, and from the long line of prophets whose words had echoed through generation after generation? And he trusted the music heard in the sacred edifice, although it might die away within its walls, would yet ascent like incense to the throne of the Most High.

And would it not also be a temple of justice? Within its walls would be declared those principles from which all human laws must derive their origin, and have authority. Here, also, would be declared that divine Decalogue emanating from God himself, written by His finger, and delivered to His prophet. Moreover, within these walls would be pronounced the inevitable sentence which would follow the transgression of man – the punishment of sin – but for the consolation of man, it would also be declared that justice will be "tempered with mercy" and pardon will be given to those who repent of their transgressions through the atonement of the Redeemer of mankind.

And would it not be a regal residence, inasmuch as they had good ground for hope that when two or three were gathered together within those walls for the purpose of solemn prayer, He would condescend to vouchsafe His spiritual presence amongst them, to listen to their supplications? It would be a holy and divine audience temple for the Most High, who would not dwell in earthly tabernacles, for the whole world is His, but He would be present amongst humble worshippers in their faithful supplications. It would therefore be, in the true sense of the word, a regal residence, the habitation of Him by whom kings reign, and a hall of audience for Him who is from everlasting to everlasting King of Kings, and Lord of Lords. He trusted that it would be considered by all who had participated in that work in that they had enjoyed a great privilege, a privilege for which they should be right thankful to God that He had put it into their hearts to rebuild for Him a house of prayer.

Many associations were connected with the erection of that place of worship, which they had determined to raise in the place of the more ancient one, and he trusted that all who participated in the work might be blessed with the promise held out in the gospel- and they that be of Thee shall build the old waste places; thou shalt raise up the foundations of many generations; "and though shalt be called the repairer of the breach – the restorer of paths to dwell in".

And to that he hoped, unlike many who were called to assist in building the ark and were never permitted to enter its walls of safety, they would be blessed in the art and in its result. He would only further hope that every success might attend that good and great work. As should only do so by the blessing of God; for though Paul might plant, and Apollos water, God alone could give the increase. Might His Word increase through the ministrations performed within those precincts and in the prayer of the Scriptures He would earnestly **hope that "those who were planted in that house of the Lord might flourish in the courts of the house of their God".**

The Rector then briefly addressed the assembly. He said he felt most happy that the commencement of a new church had happened during his incumbency, and he might add that he thought there was not an inhabitant of the parish who did not experience the same feeling in a greater or less degree. He would ask of them to let that event be the commencement of a new and brighter era for the parish of Bucknall.

They all knew that, for many years, the old church had been notorious, but he trusted its notoriety had now come to an end, and that a new and better state of things would arise. He trusted that Bucknall, for the future, instead of being a bye-word and described as a dirty place, might be an example to other places in the neighbourhood.

After three hearty cheers had been given for the success of the undertaking the assembly dispersed. The workmen were afterwards entertained at a substantial dinner, at the Red Lion Inn, at the expense of the church wardens and some of the parishioners.'

"That's it. I can breathe now. Very religious, very uplifting. Shame you weren't working on it John, you could have got a free lunch."

"Nah, eet's tay much loik a court rooem. Dost nah, thee 'olds preesoners theer, in thut lettle cottage o'er rowd, opposeete? Theer's an ondergrun tunnel laydin' tot pub – thee brengs preesoners through tonnel tot pub fer theer 'earing wi' mojestreete."

"Talking about magistrates, I wonder what Job Meigh thought, being overlooked to do the laying of the cornerstone, with Smith-

Child being chosen instead – I mean, Smith-Child isn't even from Bucknall and Job Meigh, a renowned magistrate, only lives over the road. You'd think they would have asked Mr Sneyd, also, though, as he donated the land?"

"Yer, Job Meigh dinna looek too 'appy, 'specially as 'e wus ont' building commettay en 'is son, William, wus ilected Cheermon. Ded yer knah too, thut Job Meigh 'ad doneeted £100 towods belding custs asaydes frum advancing monney to paye the belder during the corse o' cunstruction? Mind -, eet wus a greet sarvice - a blissing ont' chorch. Com te thenk o' it, nah, thee 'ad te git an Anglican en Job Meigh wus stell a prominent mimber o' the Bethesda Methodist New Connexion Chapel, at thus tarm, in 'Anley, so 'e wutna bay up fer it."

"Yes, Job Meigh is actually buried at St Mary's Church. After the building of the new St. Mary's Church in Bucknall, he became more involved with the Anglicans and changed his affiliation. He purchased the most prominent spot by the chancel for a family vault. His wife's there too, along with William, you remember, he died in 1876. I believe he was 69. I don't know why Elizabeth allowed herself to be buried alongside Job, but she did and I suppose she didn't want to be extricated from being, eventually, with the rest of her family. Also, as I told you a couple of days ago, Job was still haunting Ash Hall, so she was never really rid of him, so might as well be with him after death.

I heard about the forthcoming funeral for Job Meigh – it must have been late January or early February 1862 - and went along –

I don't know why – probably to make sure the old blighter was actually buried." We both laughed at that.

"Yer, ah saw th'obituary thut appayred int' Staffordshire Sentinel. Ah wint alung te sey th'earse but stooed itesayde, dinna go in."

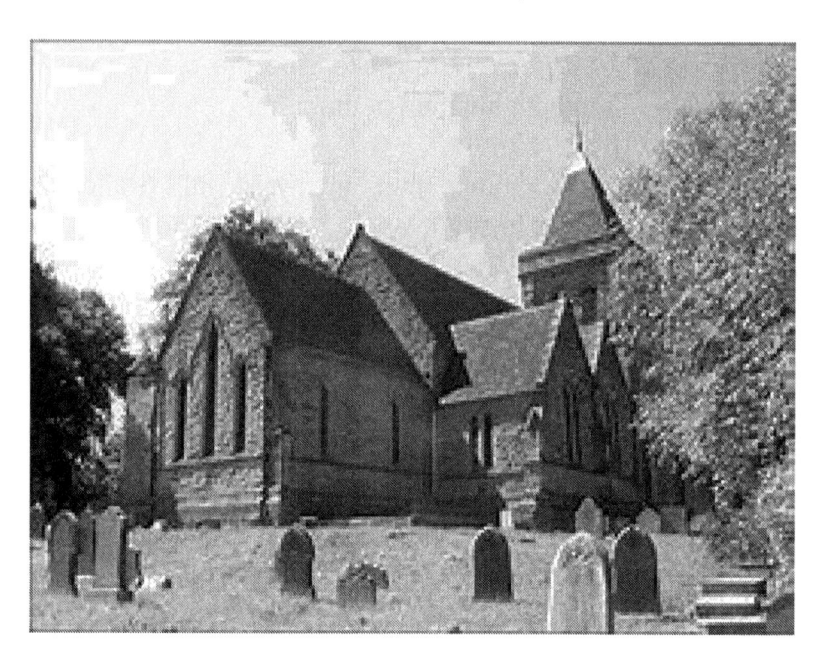

St Mary's Church, Bucknall

"Well, you know me and my record-keeping. I've got the obituary, if you give me a minute…….. there, dated 8 February 1862. It reads:

'Our obituary last week contained a notice of the death of this gentleman, who, although of late years he resided in comparative seclusion, and was seldom seen in public, formerly occupied no insignificant position in the district and took no small share in public affairs.

Mr Meigh was one of the original trustees of the Hanley market, and with his death the last of the original trustees of that property has passed away. He took an active part in the erection of the present market and the Town Hall at Hanley, and in developing the resources of the trust. He was a Deputy Lieutenant of the County and county magistrate, but for four or five years before his death, took no active part in magisterial business.

In the riots of 1842, Mr Meigh did good service in the cause of law and order, and while he took up the firm position which his character as a magistrate rendered necessary, he did not lose sight of the utility of a use of the "milder art" of persuasion, and to good purpose. Mr Meigh was associated with the late Mr Ridgway in the development of the then young cause of Methodist New Connexion, and in founding the spacious edifice belonging to that body in Albion Street, which the deceased gentleman attended up to a recent period. Beside the liberal support he afforded to the Connexion, Mr Meigh extended substantial sympathy to many other objects of piety, of philanthropy and charity. He was, in early life, a member of the late well-known firm of Hicks, Meigh and Johnson, china manufactuers at Shelton, and at the dissolution of the partnership he retired with an ample fortune.

While in business he was more than once honoured by medals from the Society of Arts for improvements in the ceramic art, and took great interest in all attempts to preserve the health of the class of workmen called "dippers", by trying to dispense with the deleterious ingredients in the compositon of the glazes. His well-known probity and business ability led to his occupying positions of great trust, among which we may mention the duty of winding up the affairs of Sparrow and Nickisson's bank at Newcastle, in 1825 or 1826, and afterwards the executorship under the will of the late Thomas Kinnersley, Esq., the well known banker and iron master.

Mr Meigh died at his residence, Ash Hall, near Hanley, on Tuesday week at the advanced age of 78 years. The remains of the deceased gentleman were interred in the family vault in Bucknall churchyard, on Thursday. The funeral, like the life and character of the deceased, was unostentatious, but a number of Mr Meigh's friends, and also his tenants, accompanied his remains to their resting place. The cortege consisted of some twelve or thirteen carriages, conveying the friends of the deceased, and of his tenants, who walked.

The following was the order of the procession:

Carriage containing the Rev. T Rider, the Rev. W Longbottom, and the Rev. J Coulton .
Carriage containing J M Blagg, Esq, and Thomas Goddard, Esq
Carriage containing J W Ward, Esq, W Ridgway, Esq and J W Pankhurst Esq.

THE HEARSE
Mourning coach containing W Meigh, junior, Esq., W M Meigh, Esq, W Brownfield Esq and Thomas Peake, Esq.

Family Carriage
Carriage containing Sparrow Wilkinson, Esq., R Wright, Esq., and Joseph Clementson, Esq.
Carriage containing Mr J Watkin, Mr S Cole, Mr W Bates and Mr R Bates
Mr Meigh's tenants.

The Rev. C H Heath, Rector of Bucknall, performed the funeral sevice.
The arrangements of the funeral were entrusted to Messrs Bate & Son, and Mr J Watkin, of Burslem.'

Of course, you will have noticed, John, there was nothing about injuring his wife for life. They wouldn't say that at a funeral – they only mentioned things he was recognised for and, funnily enough, nothing at all about his family.... Oh, John, I've just noticed, Elizabeth Meigh is not even mentioned as being in any of the carriages. Oh crikey – she didn't even go to his funeral!"

"Shay cod've bin seek. Eet wusna lang efter thut, abite a yayre, thut shay 'ersen dayed."

"Possibly. I hadn't been in touch with her for some time. But, I still like to think she'd stayed away out of protest. Good for you, Elizabeth, if you did!"

"Yer, 'e wus a bougre."

"Looking at this obituary again, John, I notice that there were a few people I knew, who were at that party Job Meigh had organised in 1842, and who were on the board of magistrates at the Pottery riot meetings I attended – Mr Sparrow Wilkinson, Mr Joseph Clementson and William Brownfield were at the party. Thomas Sparrow Wilkinson is another renowned potter – his family is mentioned in Burke's peerage, 'don't you know' – that was one of his set phrases, a real toff. Joseph Clementson owned the Phoenix Works at Shelton and was another member of the Bethseda New

Connexion chapel. William Brownfield owned the Wood and Brownfield pottery. He was a Whig and member of the Bethseda New Connexion too. He was originally from Carrigill in Cumberland. He came to the Potteries in 1811, probably when he was about 17 or so. He worked first as a collier, then apprenticed himself to J & W Ridgway and by 1832 was able to set up his own business at the Phoenix Works, Shelton, in partnership with Jonah Read, until the partnership ended in 1839, when he carried on on his own. He'd managed to get over to Canada where he set up a successful export business to Canada. So, he did very well for himself.

"Ay, tokking abite funerals, dost rimember funeral o' Hugh Bourne? Eet wus in '52. 'E'd leeved at Ford Hayes Ferm, just rayght off Clough Rowd. 'E wus a Premetive Methodist, following Weslian mithods en used te praych int' open eer. 'E wus well loved rind 'ere. Thee aven accipted women praychers, wud yer nah! Onyweeys, 'e dayed on 11th October 1852 en 'is funeral wus attinded bay 16,000 payple!"

CHAPTER 17 – CHANGE HAS COME

I was making lunch for us both the next day and worrying why we hadn't heard any news from the pit. I didn't want to bring this up with John, it would do no good anyway. What would be would be. I suppose they were waiting for the water to subside before they could get into the far reaches of the pit. Maybe they had to dam up the water flowing in from the stream that flooded the pit, which was probably taking time, before they could start pumping out the water.

I had to occupy my mind with something else, and as we were having lunch, started talking about all the things that had happened, generally, since the riots of 1842, the year John and I met. John mostly just listened as I talked – just adding a few "ums" and "ahs" and "ah rimember thut" and butting in when he had something to say. He had never been a great talker anyway, but was a good listener.

"You know, we've come a long way since 1842, John, the political reforms and inventions. The Chartists didn't disappear after the riots. They were still campaigning, and in 1860 The Reform League, led by John Bright and former Chartists were still actively trying to get manhood suffrage, the vote for men. It wasn't until the Reform Act of 1967 that urban working men were at last given franchise. Then it wasn't until 1872 that secret voting was introduced So, four out of the six requests in the People's Charter that the Chartists had campaigned so vehemently for, had actually come about and that had taken nigh on 30 years. The only requests still to be agreed on are Annual elections and the payment of MPs. I suppose that will come about eventually."

Of course, I knew payment of MPs would eventually come about. Annual elections were, however, probably a step too far.

"Old 'Capper' Joseph Capper, the Chartist we heard in Hanley back in 1842, was loved by the people. His arrest and imprisonment were cruel – he was an old man, an extremely pious man. He didn't take part in any of the riots, nor ever encouraged any resort to force. His words were misinterpreted and he was convicted of sedition. The belief amongst his followers was that it wasn't the judge who interpreted the law and tried him, it was the overpowering sentiment of the middle and upper classes that something must be done, that some signal retribution must be inflicted upon every man who had been at the front at the time of the riots, however sacred his motives, and however noble his endeavours to guide this movement. He'd been a blacksmith and, if I remember correctly, a quote about him read, 'A purer and a more loyal patriot did not live in the Queen's realms than Old Capper. A more God-fearing and man-loving man could not be found in the whole area of the British dominions. Yet this venerable man was taken from his peaceful home and quiet industry as if he were a murderous villain.' He commanded such respect because he had never raised a finger against anyone or anyone's property. He was able to prove that he did not incite people to get pikes and torches, but his proof was not believed because the rich and powerful wanted someone to blame. He had brought witnesses to Stafford and had kept them there for a fortnight to prove that the witnesses against him were liars. Unfortunately, the witnesses were obliged to return home as Capper's case wasn't heard til last, and his money had run out. This misfortune deprived the old man of the evidence of those who knew him well, and who knew what he had said and done. He was tried and sentenced to two years' imprisonment for sedition. He had only served six months when, again, in 1843, he was put on trial for conspiracy, along with Cooper and Richards. However, he had suffered so terribly in prison, being seriously ill. He said that the prison diet of skilly had 'scoured' his inside – which it is known to do.

For 30 years he had tried in his humble way, to do his religious preaching, and had never received a sixpence for his service. He thought it wrong that men had not votes instead of houses. He was getting old himself but he wanted to leave the world better than he found it. He had a poor, aged wife, who had gone with him through all his troubles, and whom he esteemed more than all the world. At his trial he stated that he knew nothing of the proceedings of Cooper, Richards and Ellis, nor had he joined them in any conspiracy. Of course, a verdict was given against him. A sentence of acquittal would have been a miracle of simple justice in such a time and with such a jury; but, though virtually acquitted on his second trial, the injustice done him on his first trial was carried out. He served his two years in Stafford Gaol and, at the end of the time came out broken down in health, but strong as ever in the consciousness of his integrity. He was met as he came out of Stafford Gaol by a few friends and he went on his way home through the Potteries, triumphantly applauded by thousands, who believed in his perfect innocence of the charge for which he had so cruelly suffered. In all the years of his life, after this, no man in Tunstall commanded more regard and honour and reverence. He told men, who were driven to madness by their wrongs, neither to injure any other man nor destroy his property. He urged them to be sober and industrious. He urged them to carry forward their noble work, to make their country great and free and good. He was a workman who believed labour to be worship. He was a neighbour who believed in charity. He was a patriot who believed the good of his fellow-countrymen was the surest source of their welfare and strength. He was a citizen who saw the greatness and glory of his country must spring from its freedom, its industry and its character. Such were his ideals. For all this, his country banned him, denounced him and imprisoned him. His kindliness, his rugged manliness, though now softened by suffering and long experience, won for him a unique position in the esteem of all who knew him."

"Oh, thut's a sed stury."

"Yes, he died in January 1860, but I can see something of him in you, John – not the religion, but sober and industrious. You want to see your country great, free and good and relish in the work that man can create and you help anyone who needs it."

"Ah, but ah'm no a forgeeving sert. Ef ah'm 'urt, ah'm 'urt fer a lang tarm. Eet's a sert o salf-prutection."

"Yes, I know……. Anyway, I have a bit more you might be interested in about Joseph Capper."

"Olraight, yer've go may ottintion."

"It was 1850 and the Pope had issued a Bull giving territorial titles to Roman Catholic bishops in this country. Everyone was up in arms.Meetings were held all over the country, denouncing the Pope. One meeting was held in Tunstall, in a church school in the autumn. Clergymen and even Wesleyan and Primitive Methodist ministers were invited. The meeting was crammed with enthusiastic opponents of the Church of Rome. The people did not know then that it was the recent developments in the Church of England itself, which had led the Pope to that act of aggressiveness so widely resented. Torrents of abuse against the Pope were wrought. Old Capper rose, amid loud and long-continued applause. The old man stood with beaming face and shining silvery hair. Those ringing cheers were intended to convey more than approval of his present function. They were the triumphant endorsement, on the part of most there, of the noble and patriotic life he had lived.

Here was a man,who, eight years before, had been sentenced to imprisonment for sedition, against whom it had been solemnly sworn that he wished to destroy the Church of England, and yet this same man, six years after he had come out of Stafford Gaol, was received by clergymen and magistrates and the representatives of all the 'respectable' people in the town, standing and applauding the old man. When this striking and signiifant ovation was over, the venerable man said a few simple and earnest words, conveying more than any oratory heard that evening in defence of the faith once delivered to the Saints.

Then, holding up in one hand a copy of the Pope's Bull, and taking in the other hand a candle from the table, he applied the flame to the lower part of the paper. This flame suddenly rose, and so did the cheers of the people. The old blacksmith's hand never shrank from the thin flame of the paper. This was held till the last shred of it fell in a feeble flicker from between his finger and thumb. This was Old Capper's last famous appearance in the town."

"Yer, ah've 'eerd thut stury afore. Mar nipheuw, Charlie, fer Tunster, tolt it may. So poignant and moving."

"Yes, and I met up with a young man who told me the story. He came from Tunstell too and had been a potter since the age of seven. His family had been put in the workhouse at one time, after his father was trying to defend the rights of the workers for more pay. His father's boss ensured that the boys father would get no work anywhere else. He had a hard life. They got out of Chell workhouse 'The Bastille' eventually and he managed to get work as a toy-maker in Burslem, through a friend of his father's. I met him when he came to visit his mother, who had been admitted to the hospital. It's a story you don't easily forget."

Anyway, we'd finished lunch and went into the garden to get a bit of sun.

We can have a sort of game. A memory game. Let's see who can name all the inventions and happenings that have come about since 1842. Are you up for it?"

"Ah dunno, but ah'll gee it a tray."

"Ok, I'll start. Oh, if you win, I'll make supper, if I win, you can buy me a pint..... I believe in July 1844 the national conference in the Temperance Hall in Burslem decided to hire a legal advisor, W P Roberts – known as the miners' attorney. He defended miners in court but he was up against a brick wall, that had to be smashed down and rebuilt - the legal system itself. New laws needed to be made and approved by Parliament. The Union established a general fund to support all miners on strike. – so this was the beginning, no matter how frail, of a start to permanent trade unions. Oh, and talking about the legal system, in 1880, a court of Quarter Sessions was set up.

Oh, and in 1857 Hanley and Shelton became a borough – the Borough of Hanley."

"Thut's two thengs, yer no geeing may a chonce."

"Ok, sorry, your turn."

"Raight, yer knahs ah loik mar reelweey 'istory - frum 1864 Stocke 'ised the repeerr shups o the North Staffordshire Reelweey en Kerr Stuart & Co Ltd, th'independent reelweey locomotive manufacturers 'an tacken up residence theer, just thus yeyre. Beesically, ol o' Britain's cuvered bay reelrowds neow. Way con himport en hexport to ol o'r the wereld."

"I didn't know that, thank you John." though, naturally, I knew the railway was one of John's interests.

"Ah've go sommit else, as you 'ad two goss. In 1870 a borough fayre brigeede wus hestableeshed, at lest, olthow the brigeede were requeered te act as spicial constables whun nicissary. Ah telt yer thut as way was going ryned Etruria te say th'official 'cutting o' the sod' cirimony, tacking pleece in a fayld, fer the neuw reelweey - rimimber whun the gayzer brok 'is selver speede."

"Yes, that was a laugh..... and, on the same subject, I believe, Stoke-on-Trent railway station was opened, in October, 1848, by the North Staffordshire Railway Company."

"Ah, thus mint thut Trent en Mersey Conal, built 60 yayrs arlier, lust allov eet's treede. Cleey cod bay hemported much queecker bay reel. En, of coss, the six tines sterted to grer wi' mer payple comming in. Bursley, the 'muther tine' wus steel lurgest thow."

And there have been so many inventions since 1842. Morse developed his electronic telegram in 1844. That has meant that ships can contact ships at sea, and messages can be sent from one country to another, using his dots and dashes to represent the letters of the alphabet."

"Int 1840s Elias Howe wus the fost Amirican to hinvint a seuwing machine. Olso thus dickeede so th'envintion o' the fost vulcanaized rubber pneumatic tire, the fost green iliveetor, en the fost steepler."

"Anesthesia and antiseptics date to this decade, as does the first dentist's chair. Oh, Jane Eyre was published in 1847. I did enjoy reading that, although it did cause a bit of a stir here with her talk of fidelity, hypocrisy and Rochester's numerous liaisons. By the by, I even heard that Charlotte Brontë even attended one of the Chartist speeches."

"Charles Goodyear pattented his volcanised rubber band in 1845. That must be so useful in machinery." ....So, I thought to myself, one day soon, I might even get my washing machine!!

"In 1845 new tine 'all wu opened in Fountain Square en police steetion moved theer."

"Chloroform was a Godsend. First used by James Young Simpson as a general anesthetic during childbirth. Prominent churchmen objected to it, quoting Genesis 'God intended women to suffer pain during childbirth' – poppycock, Queen Victoria soon showed them what for by requesting its use during her labours. The safety pin has also been invented. That was such a boon to women trying to tie their babies' nappies."

"In 1847 Th 'Anley County Court District was histableeshed – eet originally covered th'ole of Potteries wi' the court mayting at 'Anley Tine 'All."

"Joseph Lister, a Scottish surgeon, started to use antiseptic in hospital for cleaning wounds and surgical equipment and insisted his surgical team clean their hands with Carbolic Acid prior to operating. He was proved right as the number of patients who then became infected, decreased considerably and the process was adopted around the world, revolutionising medical care."

"Sa, fother aweey, in 1851 theer wus the Greet Hixebetion at Crystal Palace. Yer, eet was cunstrocted frum a casst aion freeme en glass. Ah 'eerd thut seks mellion payple attinded – abite 1/3rd o the hintayre population o Greet Britain! It olsa faytured the fost public convayniences, aich parson peeying 1 pinny te use 'em."

"Wow, that's what I call progress." I laughed.

"Thut's nowt. Elisha Otis henvinted the left. Ah've nivver sin one in opereetion en ah thenk ah mayt bay frittened to go inte one, but thee sees e' belds in an ottomeic spreng-opereeted breeke system te stup cob folling ef keeble brok."

"I'm saying nothing, (of course I wasn't going to say that lifts and escalators had always been an everyday thing in my youth)...and definitely frightening to think of a lift plunging to the ground and the people inside being killed...... but, yes, they're now building tower blocks in America, and installing Otis' lifts, which they call 'elevators' over there."

I began thinking of that awful fire at Kings Cross, in 1987, caused by a lit match being dropped, which fell down into the workings of a wooden escalator and setting fire to rubbish that had been allowed to collect there. Cigarettes were banned on the underground after that. 31 people were killed and 100 injured. No-one had been trained to deal with fires on the underground as there hadn't been one before and staff were complacent. A violent, prolonged tongue of fire, and billowing smoke, came shooting through a tunnel, that people were desperately trying to escape through to get to the ticket hall. The tunnel acted as a funnel for the flames – known as a trench effect, burning everone in its path. I was living in London at the time and I remember my dad, my real one that is, (not one I'd made up to appease Job Meigh), ringing me up to see that I was safe.

"Wek oop. Er yer deedrayming?" I heard John say. "Eet's yur tarn"

"Sorry, John. OK, let's see, yes, on the world front we had Balaclava and the charge of the Light Brigade in the Crimean War, on 25 October 1854."

"In 1855 thee belt the Panama Reelweey crussing frum th'Atlantic ol the weey o'er te Pacific. Thus lid onte the belding o' Panama Conal eetsen. Thee codna 've one wi'ite t'uther."

The telegraph, after various tries and tribulations, was developed by Samuel Morse into a recording device. He managed to create Morse code and send the first telegraph message across two miles in 1938."

"Ay, ah'm nor 'evving that. Yer said frum 1842. That's afore that tarm."

"OK, I've got another. Isaac Singer invented a sewing machine in the 50s. This attempt would be the one that would become a household name in the years to come." I remembered my mother having a Singer sewing machine. "Yes, John, I still haven't got one but I've believe ladies opposite the Windmill have got one and are making clothes for sale. As you know, before that, those old ladies were sewing everything by hand and families had to sew clothes using a thread and needle. The sewing machine, as far as I know, wasn't a new invention – various people had tried since a double-pointed needle was invented back in 1830 – this, it seems, eliminated having to turn the needle after every stitch."

"Olraight, ah've gor anuther. Pullman treen slayping ker, neemed efter eets henvintor, George Pullman."

Footsteps in the Past – The Secret

"Good, John, and Louis Pasteur developed pasteurization, a momentous scientific advance."

"'Enry Bessemer diviloped 'is convarter in 1857. Prayviously stayl 'ad bin too ixpinsive te produce, en wus onnly used in smo, ixpinsive atems, sich as knoives, serds en earmour."

"Yes, I believe Bessemer had a problem due to the impurities in the iron and, despite spending tens of thousands of pounds on experiments, he could not find the answer. Bessemer was sued by the patent purchasers who couldn't get his patent to work. In the end Bessemer set up his own steel company because he knew how to do it, even though he could not convey it to his patent users. Bessemer's company became one of the largest in the world and changed the face of steel making."

I continued, while John was trying to think of something else. "Of course, we can't forget the Indian Mutiny of 1857. The Indian Mutiny against British rule in India had been begun by Indian troops (sepoys) that were in the service of the British East India Company. The revolt began when the sepoys had refused to use the new rifle cartridges they were given, which were rumored to be lubricated with grease that contained a mixture of pigs' and cows' lard (and as such would be impure to the Hindu and Muslim troops that used them). The refugees were shackled, and their fellow soldiers had used this as an excuse to shoot their British officers and march on Delhi. On March 29th, the sepoy Mangal Pandy of the 34th Native Infantry refused orders on the parade ground at Barrackpore, and he was hanged. Thereafter the mutineers were known to the British troops as 'pandies'. The earlier massacres were overshadowed by what took place at Cawnpore, where General Wheeler commanded a small garrison that was defending the approximately 330 women and children that had been in the city. Having negotiated safe passage out of Cawnpore with Nana Sahib, Wheeler took his force and dependents down to the river Ganges and into the waiting boats. The embarkation was brought under heavy fire. Only one boat escaped, but Wheeler and most of the soldiers were killed, leaving only some 200 women and children to be taken prisoner. When news reached the rebels of an approaching relief force they massacred the prisoners and threw their dismembered bodies into a well, which became and remains the cause célèbre of the Mutiny."

"1859 saw William Smith drelling 60ft dine en descuvering ile in Pennsylvania. Theer gitting ite abite 20 barrels a deey neow. Thus wus the fost ile tacken frum ondergrun. Afore thut thee cod onnly collict ile thut 'ad bobbled te sofface inte pooels. No-one kneuwe whut thee 'ad at fost – thee wus drelling fer wotter, funt ile en clowsed will dine. Selly suds."

"OK, in 1863 the Emancipation Proclamation was made by Abraham Lincoln on January 1st. It freed all Confederate slaves. This had followed from the statements he made after the 1862 Battle of Antietam. He was not able to declare from within the boundaries of Confederate states, but from the battle lines of the conflicting armies as the commander-in-chief. It allowed the Union to recruit black soldiers (and succeeded in over 180,000 of them joining)."

"Lit's gerra way frum America. London installed eet's fost ondergrun reelweey, 'The Metropolitan Railway', betwayn Paddington Steeshion en Farringdon Strayt via Keng's Cruss.

The brunze stotue o Josiah Wedgewood, opposeete reelweey steeshion, wus iricted in 1863 en next year saw opening o' the Stocke reelweey warks o' the North Staffordshire Reelweey. Oh, en osso, Stocke Setty Fooetbow Club wus fiynded arint sem tarm." The tame wus neow beeg enogh t 'an a fooetbo club, en o 'cos o' reelweeys coming.

"You're running away there, John, with your railway and football facts. Looks like I'll be making you supper! OK, I'd better see what else I can remember. ....OK – more in your line but 1864 sees the first use of a submarine to torpedo an enemy vessel."

"Ah noss ah sid ah dinna wunt onytheng abite America, but ah sopposs eet kiynts. The Sevel Wur inded in 1865 en thun ont' 14th April Prisident Lincoln wus shut en murtally wooended bay John Wilkes Booth whayl at thayatre."

"OK, let's see.... 1866, yes, The Austro-Prussian War. The Prussian army beat the Austrian and Saxon ones. The campaign was planned by Otto von Bismarck, with the intent of unifying Germany." I don't know why I brought this up, it was just a reminder of one of the mistakes I had made why teaching, which led, to Graham's death. I hoped John hadn't remembered the link.

Obviously he hadn't, or chose to ignore it, as he continued, "Ah belayve, int' sem yayre, Alfred Nobel hinvinted daynamate."

"Yes, 1866 saw the building of The North Staffordshire infirmary."

"Oh, I've got another, I've got to catch up with you, John. Yes, in 1867 America purchased Alaska from Russia for roughly two cents per acre of land. They got a good bargain there!"

"Durring th'American Seevel Wur in 1860s, Richard Gatling peetented 'is machine gun, neemed efter 'im, en Robert Whitehead heenvented torpedo. George Westinghouse osso heenvented arr breekes, en tongsten stayle wus fost mayde."

"Ok, Alexander Graham Bell patented the telephone in the 1876, although there seemed to be a bit of a squabble over rights to the patent. Michael Faraday was the first person to contribute to the idea of a telephone when he proved that metal vibrations could be converted into electric impulses. However, it seems that a device needed to be invented that could convert sound waves, which Philip Reis managed to achieve in 1861. The invention of a practical telephone is credited to Alexander Graham Bell and Elisha Gray, who worked on their projects independently. The invention became a reality on March 10, 1876, when Bell transmitted the first sentence through his simple phone, 'Mary had a little lamb.'"

In the 1870s, Thomas Edison invented the phonograph and the lightbulb and the first-ever movie was made. Also, in 1867, although we already had the printing press, Christopher Sholes created the first reliable typewriter for personal use. He licensed the patent to Remington and sons from New York. Also, I believe I read that Thomas Edison built the first electric typewriter in 1872. That's great, isn't it? There they are making electric typewriters and we haven't even got electricity in our parish, let alone any of the six towns!"

"Nah, way're olweeys at th'end o' queue!"

"Getting closer to today, Stoke on Trent Municipal Borough was created in 1874."

"En gerring beck te fooetbow – Port Veele Fooetbow Club wus hestableeshed in 1876."

"Anyway, so, this was our industrial revolution set ready to roll. We've gone from hand production methods to machines, new chemical manufacturing and iron production processes, the increasing use of steam power and water power, the development of machine tools and the rise of the mechanised factory system as well as the rise in population of towns and cities. …. So, who won? Do I make tea or do you take me down the Red Cow?"

"Ah thenk eet wus a taye, missel, so 'ow abites way di the tway."

CHAPTER 18 – THE SECRET REVEALED

We didn't stay in the Red Cow for long. It was crowded and we were both a bit tired.

We were just about to get ready to go to our separate beds and I had just one candle lit to take upstairs with us. John was talking about when he might be ready to go back to work. He assured me he would, of course, take it easy and get the younger men to do the hard graft, taking a back-seat as supervisor. He had already been doing so, before the heart attack, but I advised him to just do half-shifts to start off with and see how he felt.

All of a sudden there was an unexpected knock at the door. We both jumped at this. Oh, I thought to myself, this could be someone from the coal mine, with the dreaded news that they'd found Alfred's body. We hadn't talked about Alfred in the last couple of days, since the disaster and John's heart attack. I deliberately didn't want to bring up the subject again and had been trying to take John's mind off it. John obviously knew this and said nothing either. Of course, it was in the back of both of our minds that we should hear some news soon, it had been dry and warm the last couple of days, so the water in the mine would have gone down.

Just as I was about to get up to open the door, a shadowy figure appeared and stood in the dim corner of the room.

I nearly fainted, and flopped back down into my chair. "Alfred, is that you?" I looked at John, he was sitting there with his mouth open, seemingly too stunned to say anything or able to move.

I got up and rushed to him, wanting to throw my arms around him, but was stopped in my tracks as he held his hands up, palms towards me. "Do not touch me mum."

"What, …. what do you mean? After all this time of worry and I can't hold you?" I could feel the salt tears beginning to roll down my cheeks. "Let me give you a hug, Alfred. I'm so pleased to see you safe and sound. We both are." looking at John.

Just then, another figure seemed to float through the door. A figure that appeared to be lit from inside – emitting a glow. A figure wearing dark trousers and a modern day nurses overall.

I put my hand to my mouth and cried a muffled scream. I heard John say, shakily, "Oo are you?.................. Whut are you? Yer look sommigh fameliar. Deed ah knoh you wunct?

In answer, the spectre replied:

"I am your own Jane, who you met in 1842, John."

There was a gasp from John but he managed to get out, weakly, ……"Spirit, please continue."

"Your wife, Jane, has been trying to explain to you over the last 40 years what actually happened to her, but you have been unwilling to listen. I don't blame you, but this led to you separating and so many good years together have been wasted. I will attempt to explain what really happened.

In our life (indicating me and herself), Job Meigh had chased you, John, on his horse, over the moors, after being enraged by what he saw as lies, connived up between the two of you, with you, John, desperately trying to avoid Job Meigh's riding whip, slashing down on you. You fell into one of the many old mine shafts and then Job Meigh rode off, leaving you to die. We had been running behind you and Job Meigh lashed his whip at us (indicating me and herself again), then went on to chase you. We were desperately crying out your name at the edge of the mine shaft but with no response. I, just me that is, then suddenly found that I was again in 2019, from whence we came, and you, John would have been long dead. I suffered a nervous and physical breakdown and was in hospital but somehow found myself walking out of the the hospital to come back to Ash Hall. I was desperately ill. We were both in limbo at this time, with me hanging on for life in 2019 and you, Jane, hanging on for life in 1842 after collapsing in Bridle Path, following the riots in Burslem. We could not survive in both eras. Either you would have died in 1842 or I would have died in 2019. Your strength overpowered me as you begged to remain in 1842 to be with John. I, therefore had to die and died here in 2019, on Bridle Path."

"Ah donna onything o' thus. Ah dosna belayve yer. Eet macks na sinse. Ah dinna daye dine a moin sheft. Ah'm steel 'ere, which yer con say fer yersen." and he stood up with arms checking himself up and down his body.

"If you will allow me to continue, John…….. Our paths split gradually, with me going to join you with the crowd of rioters outside Ash Hall. Job Meigh was trying desperately to temper the crowd's wrath. Nearby, in the Bridle Path, your Jane was dying. When I returned to 2019 after seeing you killed in the pit, we were getting further apart. I was in hospital, desperately fighting for my life. In the meantime, your Jane was being given a blood transfusion, by a doctor brought in by Job Meigh. That half of me was dying too. At that point, you came to your Jane's bedside and were so desperate for Jane to live, you professed your love for her and that you wanted to marry her. Jane, in her half delirium, on hearing this, begged to stay with you. Her plea was so desperate, it overpowered my own will to survive. I'd made by way out of hospital by then and managed to get to Bridle Path. That is where I died, in 2019. We could not both survive. Your Jane lived.

"Yer, ah rimember allov thut. Ah'd realised ah loved 'er. Shay was dying en shay wus colling ite, thut shay wunted te steey. Ah dinna onderstond eet at the tarm, but ah sopposs ah do neow. Shay wunted te bay wi' may en didna wunt te retarn te 21st sintury"

I spoke up, "So, you see, John. I am from the future. That's why I know what is going to happen. That's why I made those mistakes in the classroom. They were things I knew would happen but I wasn't well enough at the time, suffering with morning sickness, being pregnant with Geraldine, that I got confused and said things that I shouldn't have said. That's why Geoffrey got murdered."

John looked to the spectre again. "Is what Jane is saying true?

"Yes, I don't know how or why I was sent back into the past, except to throw light on why your ghost was haunting Ash Hall. But, that bit of history was wiped out. It never happened because our paths diverted. You were never killed by Job Meigh in 1842 and your bones were never discovered in 2019. Jane has made her life in the 19th century, but she came from the future."

"John thought I was a witch and left me, many years ago, before Geraldine was born. He could not get over the fact that I had got Geoffrey killed, with my made-up stories or what he saw as witchcraft, in knowing what the future held."

"Yes, that was indeed a shame, but can you not forgive her John, after all these years, now finding out that, finally, that Jane was telling the truth and is no witch."

John, in answer to this, put his arm around me and kissed me. "Cosna fergeve may, Jane. Ah've bin ignorant ol thus tarm, but ah con say neow ah wus wrung. Con way mack ominds. Is eet too leet? Ah've nivver stopped loving ye."

"I would like to, John, and I never stopped loving you."

"Sa, wadyer thenk, Alfred. Yer ma en pa are gitting beck tegither." John directed these words to Alfred, standing in the corner in the dark.

The spectre spoke again, "I have brought Alfred here to see you for one last time and to say goodbye. You cannot touch him, he is in spirit form only. His physical body has died. I have been watching over him all this time since the explosion and will now direct his spirit on the right path to spiritual fulfilment –to Azrael, who will transport his soul to be with God."

I called out to Alfred, "Please son, before you leave us, I just want to say that your father did his best to try to save you, almost killing himself in the attempt, before being dragged out himself. We feel so wretched that we could not save you. But please know that you will always be loved."

"I know dad tried to save me and I knew he wouldn't be able to. It was about 8.30am and water was coming in – too much to continue working and work was stopped. But, before I could make my way out, there was the initial explosion and I was thrown into the rockface and badly injured. I was still alive but part of the roof had come down on top of me, pinning me down. I couldn't move. I was on my own, I couldn't see a thing around me. All was pitch black, except glimmers of smouldering, stinking gob-fires up ahead. I could hear the cracking of the roof above me - the supporting timbers had broken or were burning in the flames. Any second now, the roof would come in on me and I'd be a gonner. I tried to call out but the dust fumes had burnt my throat and all I could get out was a whimper. Then the water started rising. I heard the swish and rush of water, like the tide coming in on a wave. I knew people would be back there frantically trying to get miners out, but I knew I was too far down. They'd never get to me in time. I thought of you mum and dad. I knew dad would be doing his best to get to me and I knew, mum would be busy, fretfully trying to stem the flow of tears, while working on the wounded miners who had been rescued. I knew I was dying. I knew it, positively, as if I could feel my life blood seeping through the rubble and darkness which bound me. I started to cry, desperately knowing that I would never see my family, you, Kate and my two little'uns, or daylight, ever again, as the water rose over me.

.....Then, all of a sudden there was this bright light standing by me, speaking calming words. Telling me to look into the light and not be frightened. This female form rose out of the bright light and held my hand. I had this weird feeling that I knew her and that she loved me, and I felt strangely safe. She was saying that she would stay with me to the end and to believe in God and my soul would be saved. We said a prayer together as the water rose over my head... and I took my last breath. I now realise this was your spirit, mum, with me to the end. I wasn't alone and I felt so grateful.

We said our heartfelt, tearful goodbyes to Alfred but before the spirit left with Alfred she said, "I have not come for you yet Jane, but I will be watching over you and one day we will be re-united."

Both spirits then gradually faded and disappeared.

....

The coming of the spirit, my other self, and being allowed to see Alfred for the last time and to say our goodbyes, left me reviewing my religious opinions. I had lost my faith many years ago. It no longer felt relevant to my life. Wars had been won and lost in the name of religion over the centuries – bloodshed and torture in the name of God. Science had proved there was no heaven, with no God looking over us. Most Europeans had given up on religion, with only a small pocket of stallwart believers. The Catholic church was still strong, with their devout followers, but had come into disrepute, especially in schools, and monasteries where it had been found that the monks had been interfering with the young children in their care, and the nuns were no better, with their austere treatment of unwed mothers. The Islamic breakaway terroists, were causing mayhem with their attacks and bombings – the twin towers and American/NATO reprisals. Repeated terrorist attacks on the main cities of Europe, murders and bloodshed, all in the name of their faith.

However, if you took away the human failings, the tit for tat, the fight for supremacy, the scientific findings, people still had this innate capacity to believe in something. Something to pray to, to help them in times of stress. The Jane from the future had said she was taking my son to God. I believed her, although it wasn't logical. I wanted to believe there was something after this mortal life. There must be a soul, otherwise, why were people seeing ghostly apparitions?

This belief wouldn't get me going to church. Yes, it was a place to learn the religious stories and to pray, to join the community in helping others, but God wasn't there. He was deep in our own souls, a force within us and I did believe, I don't know why, that, sometimes, with extreme effort, these internal forces could be combined in mass thought and prayer to heal or bring about some major change. It was all we had left sometimes - hope.

CHAPTER 19 – THE INQUEST

There was a Coroner's Inquiry into the circumstances leading to the explosion at the Lilydale Colliery. This was held at the Red Lion, Bucknall, by St Mary's Church on 24th May. John and I and Alfred's wife, Kate, attended.

Presiding were Mr J Booth, District Coroner, Mr Wynne, her Majesty's Inspector of Mines and Mr Sawyer, assistant inspect, attended on behalf of the Home Office. Mr Perrings, the manager of the colliery, was represented by Mr Keary. A jury had been sworn in.

The coroner was first to stand. He said that the deceased, Edward Clewlow, aged 46 and Thomas Plant, aged 28, met their deaths by an explosion on 3rd May. He understood there were several other men in the pit at the time, five of whom have not been recovered.

Mr Wynne, Government Inspector, and Mr Sawyer, Assistant Inspector were next up. Mr Wynne gave background information about the pit, stating that the colliery, which was opened about 25 years ago by Messrs Forrester, Gerrard and Hawkes, is not a very extensive one but, judging from the number of times it has changed hands, the working of it does not seem to have been a very lucrative business. Mr Enoch Perrins, the present proprietor, has been in possession for up to a year and latterly only a small number of hands have been employed.

On the day in question only 16 men were engaged in the pit and they were working with naked lights, according to the custom of the place. Mr Wynne stated, "We visited the colliery the evening of the explosion. We, indicating Mr Sawyer, and others, descended the shaft with a view of endeavouring to ascertain the best course of action to be adopted. At a distance of about 8 or 10 yards from the pit bottom, we were surprised to find the pit on fire on the opposite side to which the explosion occurred. This was in the Coxhead coal seam and the imminent danger compelled us to beat a hasty retreat. The fire seemed to have been burning for some time and, to avoid an almost certain risk of a further explosion, it was considered advisable that the working should be completely flooded."

Mr Sawyer then spoke, "I advised the owner that the workings should be flooded and to allow the water to continue to rise in order that the fire may be extinguished. This will involve a delay of several weeks before any attempt can be made to re-enter the mine and recover the bodies of the men lying in it."

I was shaken to my depths to hear this. I knew Alfred had drowned but, before the visitation, I had been hoping all along, in my heart of hearts, that Alfred had found a pocket of air and, if he had survived the explosion, would eventually be rescued. I knew it had been a silly hope, but it was a mother's hope and hope was all I had left at the time. Now, on hearing Mr Sawyer's report, I realised that, if Alfred, by some miracle, had survived, he would have been drowned by the inspectors requesting the mine be flooded. I held John's hand and he, in turn, put his other arm around Alfred's wife and pulled her towards him, in an effort to comfort her. I couldn't bear to think of him lying there, wounded, trying to keep his head above water, fighting for his life and begging to be discovered before his strength ebbed away, only to hear this woosh of water coming towards him and the last glimmer of hope extinguishing as he gasped his last breath. I felt the tears starting to flow.

As if, reading my thoughts, John said, "'E mee not 'av soffered. Fang olt on thot thowt. Way knas yer spireet wus wi' 'im to the lest. Onyweeys, way knoss 'e's seefe neow."

That was a comfort. "Yes, thanks to Jane, we have been able to say our last goodbyes, John, but oh I don't want him to have suffered."

"Jane was looking efter 'im. Shay wutna 've lit 'im soffer. Think on thut, love."

I dried my eyes while John was doing his best to comfort Kate.

The first witness to be called was Anthony Hargreaves, residing at Greenfields, Bagnall, who said he was a loader at Lillydale Colliery, and was at work there on May 3rd. Mr Hargreaves tried to speak his best English for the court, the same as all the other witnesses. Mr Hargreaves said he had been engaged there four or five months.

"On the day of the explosion I was loading for a man named Gratton, who was working at the down bank head. Gratton was one of the men killed. I had noticed the place where Gratton was working that there were two boreholes on that level, one at the head and the other at the side. I cannot say how far they were driven, nor who drove them in – though I had seen Alfred Wood (our Alfred) cutting there in the side, with a 3ft blasting drill, about a week before the explosion. These two holes were in existence at the time of the disaster. That was the middle heading. I went into the bottom road during the morning to see the water, as it was bleeding from the face of the head. The water was spurting, as though forced by pressure. There were several other men with me, and I did not see a borehole on that level. Most of the men there said they did not think there was much danger, as there was not much leakage just then. Samuel Biddulph, hooker-on, son of William Biddulph, was one of the men."

Mr Wynne interupted at this point asking Hargreaves to explain to all in the room what a hooker-on was.

"Well sir, a hooker-on strikes a hook, or hooks, at the bottom of the pit, onto the corf bows. A corf is a basket made of hazel used to transport coal and the bow is a metal bow which is fitted to the corf to hang it on the winding rope, used to move the cages or skips up and down in the shaft"

Hargreaves was asked to continue. "From there I went to the heading above to begin work. Most of the men in the pit went to look at the leakage. It was generally known that the headings were driven for water. I was in the heading above till after the explosion. The water broke in. I think it came from the north but can't say for definite. I had started up the dip when I heard a great noise. It would be about five to ten minutes from the breaking of the water to the explosion. Flame came out of the thirling, that's a connecting tunnel, sir, and met me as I ran. I did not see anybody come out of the thirling, nor did I know which thirling it was. I heard my father say to Gratton, 'The water's coming, go on Elijah'. The water came on before the explosion, which happened when I got half-way up the dip. It would be from five to ten minutes from the breaking of the water to the explosion. The water overtook me and submerged me. I was rendered insensible and was pulled out. I had seen no gas that morning, nor had I observed much during the time of my engagement at the colliery."

A Juror asked Hargreaves his reaction when he saw the leakage. Hargreaves replied that, he asked his father, "What about it?" and the reply was, "It's a thing of nothing; there is twenty yards thickness of coal."

William Biddulph took the stand, endeavouring not to use his pit dialect.

"I'd been working there for four months. I went down the pit at 6am on Tuesday. The men were working and Alfred Wood, the fireman, was in the north level. At 8.30am Wood called me and said there was as much water as they could do with and there were a few droppers on the head side. I ordered the work to be stopped. I told the men to leave and came out of the pit and saw Mr Perrins, who was on the bank. I told Mr Perrins there was a sup of water, that had stopped the men working and he wanted to know what must be done. The explosion happened while we were talking. Mr Perrins started giving instructions as to what had to be done, as there was no certificated manager."

George Deville, a Waggoner, was asked to speak. "I was on my way to the pit bottom with a load from where Eaton, Gratton and

Wood were getting the coal. I was only 15 yards from the pit bottom when the explosion occurred and felt the wind and saw dust and smoke, but only a spark or two of fire. The place where I was waggoning from was about 70 yards from the pit bottom. I came out of the pit with Biddulph the butty (this I understood to be a sub-contracted miner, paid by the load, rather than by the hour)." On further questioning, Deville said the miners were using naked lights and had seen no gas in the pit nor had he heard anyone say they had seen gas.

John Marshall Holiday, certificated colliery manager, Hanley took the stand. "I was on the spot about half an hour after the explosion, and went down the pit, where I rescued Hargreaves, 59½ yards down the dip. The man was in the water. I sent him up, and then went to the edge of the water, which, by this time, had risen three yards. I then ordered all the men out. In all I rescued four men.

Arthur Robert Sawyer, Assistant Inspect of Mines for the district, presented a report as to the causes and effects of the explosion. During the management by Mr Perrins he had been in the mine eleven times. On January 21st, owing to information he had received as to the existence of fire, when he found one of the heads worked with naked lights, but there was no gas, and he could find no trace of fire. He was told that fire had occasionally broken out about ten yards from the bottom, where it could and would be watched. On March 17th he again visited the pit and, knowing that the mine was a gas-making mine, he sent for Joseph Biddulph, and warned him to use lamps at the first indication of danger. The ventilation, generally, he found good. The headings were driven with entire disregard for the 9th rule of the Mines Regulation Act of

1872, which provided that, where a place was likely to contain a dangerous accumulation of water, the workings approaching such place should not exceed eight feet in width, and that they should be constantly kept at a sufficient distance, not less than five yards in advance, at least one borehole near the centre of the working, and sufficient boreholes on each side. The seventh rule was also ignored, which enjoined the use of safety-lamps in all places where there was likely to be an accumulation of explosive gas. There was no doubt the water broke in at the bottom north heading. The water in the old working seemed to have been within seven or eight yards of the Cockshead level. That would make a head of water of eighty yards, and the pressure would be 104lb per square inch at the bottom of the dip, and this would be sufficient to break through a small thickness of coal, and drown the men at the bottom of the dip. It appeared that the roof at the bottom drift on the south side had fallen in more than usual, which would leave cavities where gas would accumulate, and this being forced by the inrush of water upon the lights of the men trying to escape from the water, caused the explosion.

Mr Keary questioned Mr Sawyer further and, in reply, Mr Sawyer stated that, "Fifty yards was the minimum thickness of rib which ought to be bored, and I knew it to be much more. I did not think the water could have broken through a rib of fifteen yards. I thought the places must have been nearer to the gibs than was supposed. I did not think falls of roof could have admitted the water, according to the extent of the falls spoken of by Biddulph.

The Coroner then questioned Mr Sawyer, who stated, "The symptoms spoken of by Hargreaves would show that they were very near the old workings, and that there was danger. If there had been falls, as suggested by Mr Keary, the water would have come from the south side, and from the roof, not from the coal. The thickness of the barrier between the mine and water at the time of the explosion would be about three or four feet. Had boreholes been made, the inundation would have been avoided. I attribute the explosion to the rush of water.

Henry Hales, a miner, living at Milton gave his report. He stated, "I was working at the Lillydale colliery at the time of the explosion. I went to work at 6am in the bottom level. I was driving along with Samuel Dawson and William Eaton, now dead, was behind me. I punched a hole in the bottom level, about a yard and 2inches deep, in the direction in which we were driving. I left at 9am, telling William Biddulph that it was bleeding faster from the head side. I'd notificed it when getting a bit of coal. William Biddulph told the foreman and they ordered me to go out and help Joseph Biddulph to put the fire out at the pit bottom. I got to the top of the dip when the explosion occurred. They had no bore hole until the morning of the explosion as far as I know. During the whole time I worked in that heading, there was no bore hole and nothing was done to show that they were approaching the heading."

Mr Wynne, Inspector of Mines for the district took the stand, " I had not visited the colliery under Mr Perrin's management. Mr Perrins was manager of the colliery at the time of the explosion, at his own request, and he would be responsible for keeping the boreholes. From the evidence as to bleeding on the face of the coal, I should say the rib of coal separating the men from the old working would be very narrow – very few feet. This would have undoubtedly been disclosed if the holes had been driven, in compliance with the Act of Parliament. The Cockshead seam was one that the water would come some short distance through; but being only a small heading, there would not be the same pressure against the rib, as would be the case of a larger one. The rib certainly must have been a good deal less than the statutory five yards. More care ought to have been taken with a mine of this kind than with a thinner seam, because, when it was worked there would be some pull, owing to the thickness."

On questioning William Biddulph further, Mr Biddulph replied, "When I saw the dropping, I did not bring the men out of the pit, because I did not think the water was so near. I wanted to tap the upper level before, seeing it was wet and the lower level dry, but Mr Perrins would not let me. He said we were far enough from the water and he would not allow it to be done."

Asked by the Coronor if William Biddulph had read the rules, he answered that his reading was not so good, to which the Coronor replied that he ought not to be a butty collier.

Mr Wynne continued that Mr Perrin's duty was to have seen that the boring was done, and Biddulph's to have done it. The water coming from the face, as described, should certainly have set the men on their guard. The consent for Mr Perrins to take the management was in consequence of a written communication from him, stating that Kirk had given him notice, and asking that he might be excused from appointing a certificated manager, he putting a practical man in charge, as there was no gas, and only twelve men at work. After consulting with Holiday, consent was given for six months."

Peter Kirk, the colliery manager, was requested to stand. He stated, "I had been the certificated manager at Lillydale, but left on the 9th March. At that time, the dip was down about 140 yards and No. 7 heading was driven about 24 yards. I had the superintending of driving it. They had kept a 12-foot boring in the heading. My orders were that, if damp were perceived, they were to stop. There were no side boreholes because they thought they were far enough away from the old workings. I can give no further evidence as, after that time, I had left the colliery.

Holiday was questioned again, by Mr Keary, "I had known water bleed through a 20 yards barrier, under very high pressure. The bleeding was a symptom that should have been attended to, as it was a sure sign of danger. The boreholes should have been kept in advance, with a plug for each hole.

Enoch Perrins, lessee of the Lilydale Colliery, was then interviewed. "I have been working the mine for about two years. The plans were prepared by my brother, now dead. The underground workings had been twice tested by Mr Steel, the surveyor to the owners of the property, and had been found accurate. According to that, the nearest of the levels was fifteen yards from the boundary, and was also the upper one. Borings were charged for and paid for according to the books. When I first became lessee I endeavoured, but unsuccessfully, to obtain a plan of Hawksey's workings. I expected water in the Cockshead Seam, but not much, as it was some twenty years since it was worked, and believed the effect of time should close up the orifice, especially as the level had been worked under Mr Kirk without showing water. I had bought a Tangye pump and had got pipes to convey steam to the Tangye at the top of the inset, where I was preparing to have bored the five yards borehole and, in the event of finding water, would have put in a stop-tap and sent up the water by the Tangye to the lodge prepared for it. Both the Biddulphs and the fireman, all men of experience, believed there was no danger. In the south side, near the fault, there had been extensive falls of roof. On the Monday prior to the explosion, there had been a fall, smashing fifty posts - like so many carrots. Joseph Biddulph had told me that, if a sudden fall had taken place on the day of the explosion, it would have sufficed to bring the water over the top of the coal, because the coal was very poor." Joseph Biddulph was asked to confirm this, and did so and continued saying that "From the 17th March till the day of the explosion, according to the report book, everything was safe. I had been in the pit every day since the 17th March but had seen neither gas, nor anything else except a bit of a fire on the north side of the pit bottom, not near the workings. The fire had been burning for five months, since January. Immediate steps were taken to put the fire out and these appeared to be entirely successful. It was never heard of again till two days before the explosion. Mr Perrins and I went to see it, but could find no flame, though there was a little smoke. Mr Perrins ordered me to attend to it."

When asked if Mr Biddulph thought it was safe to work with a fire so near, Mr Biddulph replied, "I saw no danger in working the colliery with a fire 10 or 15 yards from the upcast shaft. I cannot say that the word 'safe' should be applied to a pit in that state, although I did not think the pit was unsafe, with the fire where it was."

There was a bit of a reaction to this in the audience and an extended "hmmm" from Mr Wynne. The Coronor asked for silence in the room.

"Mr Perrins continued, "On the Thursday before the explosion, the level was as dry as possible, and I asked the men again on the Saturday if there was any sign of water. They said it was perfectly dry. No water was detected the morning of the accident, when about 11am William Biddulph said water was shooting out in the low level, and they must have the Tangye, but there had not been time enough to do anything before the explosion. As soon as the smoke of the explosion had subsided, I sent William and Joseph Biddulph down with lamps, a man named Plant, having got himself into the cage, said the water had burst in and reported back on the explosion."

There had rarely been more than ten men working in the mine since the latter end of February. With respect to the statement that Perrins had been fined for neglect, Perrins' representative, Mr Keary, replied that it was for what was supposed to be an "old pit"

The Coroner then asked Mr Perrins further questions. In reply, Perrins stated, "A fall on the south side would have admitted water from the Hawksey's old workings, by the fault. Had not the explosion happened, the Tangye would have been worked next day. I had never had any experience of water, but both Biddulph and the fireman, had thought a bore-hole of four or five feet, was quite enough. I had seen the boring on the Thursday prior to the explosion. There were boring tools that would go five yards in the pit. A six-foot drill was put in the hole in my presence. I could not say whether the fireman had the boring rods in that level. I thought six foot was quite enough of a bore with a fifteen foot rib, according to the distance. The workers were away from the boundary and, in my opinion, strengthened by my experience in the bottom workings, I gave instruction not to mine a yard without a bore, but not to mine further than five yards, as I interpreted the words of the rule 'approaching' old working as 'approaching nearly'."

Richard Wynne, mining engineer, added that it was quite possible that the theory of the water coming over the fault, and through falls in the roof, was quite possible under the circumstances.

In reply to queries by Mr Wynne and the Coroner, Perrins stated that, after the evidence as to the leakage, it was probable that some water would break in there and that a five yard borehole would have shown the danger.

The Coronor then adjourned the hearing until 21st June to enable Barlow, one of the injured men, now in the infirmary, and others to give evidence and to enable efforts to be made to recover the bodies still in the pit.

John, Kate and I returned at the later date to hear evidence from Anthony Barlow, William Tabbinor, George Philips and Henry Johnson.

George Philips looked in a sorry state and was shaking and coughing violently. He was the one suffering from after-damp, breathing in a mixture of carbon dioxide, carbon monoxide and nitrogen. Most people do not survive and I didn't think any of them would recover enough, mentally, to go down a pit again, having been so near death, but what else could they do? Their testimonies did not add much further to the trial apart from Anthony Barlow, who had suffered burns and had newly returned from the infirmary. He gave a description of the explosion, stating the the whole mine was instantly illuminated like lighting and there was a roaring whirlwind of flaming air, with heaps of ruins shaken from the roof and thundering to the shafts, with a thick cloud of coal dust, stones and timber being hurled in full force, searing his lungs as he was trying desperately to escape through the ever-rising water. He stumbled and fell into the flood and was so relieved to feel himself being hauled out and finding himself, eventually, at the surface, so grateful to his saviour and thankful for being alive.

Henry Johnson, the boy, looked a lot smaller than he should have done for his age, although wizened, as did all of them. All the miners I had seen had some distortion of their skeletal forms, bent back, knock-knees, feet bent outwards, all signs of years in the mines, with extremely long hours, and hard work, bent double and not enough food.

William Tabbinor, engine tender, spoke next. He was still heavily bandaged. He had been pulled out after nearly drowning. "I was in the pit at the time of the explosion. I had gone with Philips to connect some pipes to the Tangye pump that was being brought down and I had been there for about half an hour when I heard a loud bang and there was a big flame that came from down below. I was badly burnt and Philips has since died of his burns."

William Biddle, a pit fettler, gave evidence of finding the dead body of Edward Clewlow, about sixty yards down the dip, after the explosion.

Anyway, this was the whole of the evidence, and the coroner, in his summing-up, stated, "Some of the workers were driving a thirling, that is, a connecting tunnel, on the north side of the south dip at a depth of about 160 yards. The possible influx of water from the old workings seems to have been anticipated and two bore holes nine feet long and an inch in diameter had been kept ahead all through the driving. However, as a precautionary measure, this was insufficient to guard against the danger. The water was tapped and it began rushing into the thirling. The force of the air current thus disturbed some gas hanging about to be driven into the naked lights and a violent explosion was the result. The water raised so rapidly that, within half an hour it had filled most of the workings. Thomas Plant, Antony Barlow and William Tabbinor were saved from drowning and taken to the North Staffs Infirmary, where Plant died the following day. George Philips was saved, unconscious from the effects of after damp. A boy named Henry Jonson was got out alive. The only dead body found was that of Edward Clewlow. Owing to the rapidly rising water, the explorers were unable to go through the working and it was thought, when they retired from the mine, they were obliged to leave behind them, Alfred Wood, Enoch Barlow, Samuel Biddulph, Elijah Gratton and William Eaton, so that, altogether, seven lives have been sacrificed. Whether they were drowned or killed by the explosion cannot, of course, be ascertained. Four of the deceased were married men and had families.

The Coronor asked Mr Perrins directly if the bodies had been recovered. Mr Perrins replied, "Unfortunatately, it will be about three months before this will happen."

There was definite reaction from the audience at this, and especially the families who had lost their loved ones. We had waited so long to retrieve Alfred's body and still had another three months wait. It just wasn't bearable.

Mr Sawyer, Assistant Inspector, added to the Coronor's summing up, in a closing speech, stating that, "In my opinion, the heading had been driven with entire disregard of the general rule of the Mines Regulation Act of 1872, which enacted that, where a place was likely to contain a dangerous accumulation of water, the working approaching such place should not exceed eight feet in width, with a bore hole not being less than five yards in advance and sufficient bore holes on each side."

Mr Sawyer continued, "The 7th general rule was also ignored, which stated the use of locked safety lamps in every working approaching any place where there was likely to be an accomulation of explosive gas. For it is well known among mining engineers that the workings often contain both water and gas. The disturbance produced by the sudden inrush of water displaced the gas, which was ignited at the bare lights of the men who were trying to escape from the water."

The Coronor then directed his attention to the jurors, "I ask you, the jurors, to consider all the reports presented to you and to return your verdict."

The jury retired at two o'clock to consider their verdict.

The jury, after half and hour's deliberation, returned a verdict of "Manslaughter" against Mr Perrins, as manager of the colliery. Mr Perrins was admitted to bail.

CHAPTER 20 – HOUSE OF COMMONS REPORT

In the House of Commons, on 13th May, Mr McDonald, Sec M.P. asked the Secretary of State if his attention had been called to the statements that the mine was carried on without a certificated manager and was on fire for a considerable time, and where at least seven persons had lost their lives. Also, the owner had been fined £30 in the past for negligence. And further, he would direct someone to attend the inquest on 24th May.

Sir W. Harcourt (Secretary of State) replied: "It is a fact the mine was carried on without a certificated manager. It is a small mine in which only 12 men are usually employed and, under these circumstances, the owner, being a mining engineer, was allowed to manage it himself. It is also true that the owner was subjected to fines and costs to the extent of £30 for negligence, some little time ago and I need not say that, if repeated acts of negligence are proved, he will be held legally responsible. The Inspector's report was so clear that he did not think it would be necessary for anybody to attend the inquest on behalf of the Home Office, except an experienced Inspector.

A meeting convened by the Mayor of Hanley (Mr J Bromley), was held in the Council Chamber Town Hall, on Tuesday evening for the purpose of taking steps for opening a relief fund for the dependant widows, children and friends of the men killed by the recent explosion of gas at the Lillydale Colliery, Bucknall.

The Mayor presided. It was stated that 4 widows and 21 children had been left by the catastrophe, 1 widow and 5 children being partially provided for by the North Staffordshire Permanent Relief Society. Up to present £63 had been collected from various sources, and from that sum, £6, 5s had been expended. A letter was read from Messrs Josiah Wedgwood and Son to the effect that they thought that, while the North Staffordshire Permanent Miners' Relief Society was so poorly supported by miners, it would be doing them no kindness, but the reverse to help them.

Mr Hampton (ex-Mayor), said that there was a great deal of improvidence among miners and the fact that their wives and children were always provided for in cases of great accidents, no doubt led many of them to become improvident. It did not seem to him the true spirit of charity to get up these extra efforts to meet the necessities of extensive calamities, as more men were killed in small numbers, by ones and twos each year, than in large numbers, and for the former, no provision whatever was made by the public. He considered it a disgrace that miners did not more generally join the Permanent Relief Society.

Mr J L Hamshaw stated that, what Mr Hampton said was quite true, but, unfortunately, the wives and children suffered and not the miners themselves, for their negligence not to join the Society. He should like to see it made compulsory for men to join the Society at the various collieries in the district. Mr Hamshaw further explained that, from £200 to £300 would be sufficient to meet the present case, and that it was not intended, ultimately, to make differences between those for whom provision was made by the

Relief Society and those totally dependent, but at first, the latter would need the most urgent attention.

On the motion of Mr Hamshaw, seconded by Mr Alfieri, a committee was appointed, consisting of the clergy, Nonconformist ministers and a number of principal residents in the district, to carry out the object of a Public Relief Fund, which it was resolved to establish. A unanimous vote of thanks to the Mayor closed the proceedings.

....

That was some decision that needed a celebration, notwithstanding the loss of our dear Alfred. At least Kate and her two children would receive some provision from the Relief Society. And what a relief! It meant she could continue to look after the children and not have to scrimp and scrape for pennies, or foster them off to whoever and find work. It would be a meagre amount, but at least they would be able to survive.

It also meant that miners would have to join the Permanent Relief Society, something they had been reluctant to do. A change was coming. A change for the better.

Translation

Page 9   "I couldn't find him. I tried."

Page 20   "Well, my love, how are you".
"I've spoken with Mr Meigh, just a quick word like, as he's out doing his magistrate work. The police and army have been rounding up the people involved in the riots. Thousands of them. They've all got to go to trial. The trials are mostly taking place in Newcastle, except for the Chartists, if they catch them. He'll be gone a couple of weeks or more. Anyway, he said you can stay here for the time being. You know I've been building new houses for him on the estate. Maybe we can have one of them in a bit, once we're married. There's no rush, give us time to get to know each other better. It's all been a bit of a rush, me proposing and you accepting, although I know I love you and I don't want to wait too long to get married. What do you say to spring, you don't want a winter wedding, do you? It would give us time to build the house, make it as you'd like it, running water and all that. What do you say?"

Page 21   "I don't know about that, my love. I don't want you working when we're married. I can provide for you, don't' fear. I wouldn't be right. And when the children come along, you'll need to be home to look after them."

"As you wish, lovely. I know you do things differently down south and I would not want you to be unhappy, but I need a wife, who will be there for me and the children... when they come. I suppose, as long as you love me, we can work things out."

Footsteps in the Past – The Secret

"All right, my lovely. Get your sleep. We'll work things out."

Page 36: "He well deserved that. It was he who made the crass remark about how we poor people should use grass and leaves to make tea if we couldn't afford to buy it from the shops. Good riddance to him, that's what I say."

Page 49: "Oh, the bailiff was going on about not remembering my name as he hardly sees me there. Well, I gave him a look, as such – I didn't want to touch him, or he'd have given me a hiding, but I was angry. I mean, I come in like everyone else, when I feel like it. We're all the same. It's the way it is. Anyways, I was angry and picked up a plate someone had just finished, and smashed it. Of course, the man, who'd just finished the plate, just whacks me with it and I got in a fight with him. The bailiff just looked on – he didn't stop us."

Page 50 Jimmy continued, "I was surprised to see the bailiff there. I mean, he hardly ever comes round. I thought I'd be able to sneak in. I mean, I'd got drunk the night before and could not get out of my bed. I just thought I'd come in, do my bit, and make up for it the next week."

"Yes, it's like that everywhere. You ask anyone, you come, do your bit, and go. We have a few arguments and fights – that's normal. There's a fight on at the market this Saturday, if you're interested. One of our lads is a prize boxer, so we're all going to back him up. There's a cup as well for the winner... and prize money. It's a big thing here in the Potteries."

Page 51   "Oh, I don't know about that. No-one checks. We just get paid each week. That's all I know. I might go in on Wednesday and work over hours to catch up though.

Page 52   Jimmy continued as I bandaged his wounds. "'Because, if the Master should pay us a visit, we all look as if we're working hard. We give a kick to the drunks falling asleep at their tables. Someone will whistle if they see the Master coming and we put on a show, all quiet and industrious. He never says anything anyway – not normally anyway – just passes through, with his hands tucked at the back, under his tailcoat. Don't get me wrong – we don't want to come to his attention. I mean, he's the Master. If I'm thrown out, I'll never get a reference for anything else. I take my cap off to him and no other."

Page 53   I don't know about that, miss. I'm a Methodist and we Methodists think they're the devils work. I couldn't go against the church now, could I? They know best, miss. I'm a good Methodist. I cannot write much but I can read the Bible."

Page 62   . "I can't Jane, I'm just so, so, sore."

Page 64   "What are you fiddling with?"

"I don't want to bother you, but can you get a message to William Meigh please, that I cannot work. Tell him I'll be on my feet again soon.."
Page 65   "Have you heard anything about Alfred, Jane? Has anyone come with a message?"

'Don't fear, Jane. What will be will be? We can only hope."
"You're right, this bed's as hard as a door."

"'Ay, lass, don't get yourself so worked up."

Page 66   "Yes, we'll see, Jane. I know. I know you too, especially all that you've done for me. You've saved my life! I wouldn't be here without you, Jane. That's for sure."

"As it happens, I'm beginning to feel a bit better. Maybe I could try again to get myself up"

"Yes, good riddance – I won't come knocking on you again, door, never fear, you've done your duty, now be off with you."

"Thank you, Jane. I could eat a man off his horse, including the saddle."

Page 69   "Alright,"

Page 94   "Oh nurse – I'm pregnant again. We're starving as it is and crowded out, and I'm so weak and tired. I can't have another baby. What am I to do? Is there nothing you can do to get rid of it for me? I mean, I've only just had a baby and my husband has brought in his brother's two children and wife to live with us, and she's not working either. They're just living off us. I don't blame him – his brother died down the main and the wife's sick and cannot manage.."

Page 95   Mrs Jones continued, "We do our best. And our daughter, May, follows the local coal carts, trying to knock pieces off to bring home. The carter never says a word, as she'd have a go at him. George and I, well we try to get a few coppers some of the time, busking outside the factory gates."

"Begging my pardon for my language, nurse, but sod his ethics. This baby will kill us all. It's not fair, another baby year after year and no food and no money. My George doesn't get much work, just piecemeal. My girl, Hannah brings in a bit, shay's a potter – she's 12 now and my son, William – he's a young man now, he's 17 and a carter, but both my husband and young William, well they're down the pub, spending what little they earn, before I've got any. The other children, there's Mary, who's 8, George, who's 7, Alice, who's 3 – well they're all at school, then there's little Sarah, who's 2. Olive's not yet a year old. Is there nothing you can do? He just will not leave me alone. I've heard there's something called Penny Royal, that will shift a baby, but I tried when I was expecting our youngest and it didn't work. I was worried right through in case God punished me. I expected something could be wrong with my baby. Luckily she was alright."

Page 96   "I've heard too there's something called Slipper Elm, some women use that. They use a steel knight needle."

"I'll try, but sometimes, there's nothing I can do to stop him."

Page 98   He told me that the local families would get "a 'pennyworth' of chips between them all on bread a half-penny cake as a treat. "Before school we wait for the coal carts going to the potbanks. We knock pieces off the back to take home for mother's fire. Our fathers will go in the pub all day, where it's warm. Us children wait for the workers going home at night and grab any food they've not eaten or we try to get coppers by doing any errands. I've taken washing from Hanley up Birches Head Lane to Kerry, to a big farmhouse. We go miles taking errands, time doesn't count. Mother would say, 'I want you home early, take a basin, go down the Grant Hotel in Hanley, see if they've got any dripping. Three pennyworth of dripping is yummy. It oozes of the meat the toffs have for their meals – it's good stuff. You see, mother cannot afford to buy a joint to cook to get dripping from it."

Page 101   He smiled as he replied, "Oh, begging your pardon, but we have some ladies come in, who want arsenic to remove, if you don't mind my saying – superfluous hair. They also come in for rat poison and us it to kill kitchen flies." As I'd raised my eyebrows, which he interpreted as a look of interest, he continued. "Just for want of saying, do you know that all those floral wallpapers you ladies like, well the green colour is made of arsenic. That goes for the green feathers in the fancy hats they're fond of. It's used worldwide. I've heard say that we British have been accused by the French of poisoning Napoleon, by decorating his prison on St Helena with green-patterned wallpaper. Well I never! Good riddance to him. Good job done. I wouldn't be seen dead with green wallpaper – or maybe I would." And he laughed.

Page 105   "It was born dead, it wouldn't breathe. I had to hide it from the other children, I didn't want them seeing the body and getting upset. So I hid it. It's over there."

"Down there, in the well." she indicated.

Page 108   "My mum comes with me and says my cousin wanted a lad, a saggarmakers bottom-knocker. I applied for the job. My first job was to cut the cay and stack it for him. We'd got a concrete bench and I used to cut the clay with a sort of hay knife, cut it in length for the sides of the saggars. I would knock the clay solid with a mow in the iron frame. It was very hard work and you fair got a sweat on. I then went onto tile slabbing for fire grates. These are painted by the lasses but this was only summer work. No-one wants a tile grate in winter. So I go to Johnsons pot bank to find something else. I've been loading and unloading saggars, carrying the saggars, on my head with a roll between the saggar and my head. You put a roll on top to take the weight. We made them from women's stocking, wrapped round and round tightly. It takes the pressure off your head."

Page 111   "Yes, my love, you looked beautiful."

Page 112   "Did you make that up? I've never seen your parents. They never came to visit us. Are they still alive?"

"You never told me."

"But you didn't go to any funeral. Why didn't you say anything?"

"But what about his house and belongings? What happened to them?"

Page 113   "I do remember trying to ask you, now, but you changed the subject – you were secretive and clammed up, so I didn't say anything else."

Page 114   "Yes, then he hammered his thumb, oh he did yell, but he never gave up trying.."

"We feared the worse, love, not having heard anything." John added.

Page 115   "I'll get there, be sure of that. Some way or another. Don't fret."

Page 119   "Jane, we never really talked after I found out what happened. I think we need to go over everything again, before we can move on. A sort o' catharsis."

"I want to hear it all again. I need to."

Page 122   "Come on, you, get on with it".

Page 124   "So, how did you know that?" John piped up.
"So, they all thought you were a witch too?"

"You're at it again. Second World War? You're crackers, an empty minded idiot. We've not had any 1st World War let alone any 2nd World War. That's why I left you. Your empty talk and filling the children's heads with it.."

"You made such a mix-up that it had got our Geoffrey killed. It was your fault. You're the reason he's dead."

You're upsetting me. Get lost. If I could get out of here, I would."

Page 125 "So, how did he get killed?"

Page 127 "Yes, Job Meigh told me himself. He wanted to give me the sack too. So I had to get the story out of him. I was so perturbed. He said he'd only take me back if I left you, and had nothing more to do with you....... I wandered around aimlessly for a bit, I had to think it over, get my head in order. It was the hardest choice I ever had to make. But what you did, that was too much to bare. So, I went back and told him way were finished."

Page 125 "Yes, I've seen her around."
"I'm pleased she's getting on

Page 129 John interrupted, "Yes, I was interested in this too. There were two companies that promoted routes – The Churnet Valley Railway, getting a lane from Macclesfield to Derby, with a branch to Stoke, and the Staffordshire Potteries Railway, with a route from Macclesfield to the Grand Junction Railway mainline at Norton Bridge, with a spur to Crewe."

Page 130 "From what I remember, there are two companies that joined forced and Parliament approved a scheme to amalgamate with the Trent Valley Railway, which became the North Staffordshire Railway. People started calling it The Knotty. They then built the Pottery Line, to run from a junction with the

Manchester and Birmingham Railway at Congleton to the Grand Junction Railway at Colwich, to bring the railway to Tunstall, Burslem, Newcastle, Haley, Stoke, Fenton, Longton and Stone. The Churnet line was built to run from Macclesfield through Leek, Cheadle and Uttoxeter to join the Midland Railway line between Burton-upon-Trent and Derby, so we got a direct link between Manchester and Derby.."

"Yes, I remember, They had a roped off area for the directors and loads of other invited guests."

Page 132   Silly sods

Page 133   "Couldn't run a knees-up in a brewery".

Page 134   "Yes, it wasn't his day. After he gave his speech, it was time for him to do his fancy bit and dig into the earth to cut the first sod. From what I could see, his spade was silver in colour, made specially for the ceremony, not a proper digging tool. Trouble was, it had been so darn dry, that the spade actually buckled beneath him…. Then a gust of wind got up, and his had blew off."

Page 136   "Yes, I couldn't let her down. We'd make do, somehow or the other.

Page 137   Yes, I didn't know what to say to you. It had been so long since we'd seen each other."

"I didn't know what to get her really. I've not had much to do with young lasses."

"Bucknall and Northwood station was a bit of a time coming after that, but we got it." John added, also obviously seeing my disappointment.

Page 140   "Yes, I believe that something had just been on. A two-day gala rose show on 4th and 5th July. There were prizes given to the best competitors. And they had singers, Miss Moorland and Misters Thurnbull, Gannon, Hall and Emery, if my memory serves me right. They also had a brass and string band with dancing. I saw it advertised in the Staffordshire Advertiser.."

Page 141   "I was thinking of inviting you after Geraldine got in touch, but I thought better of it.."

John changed the subject, "They had races there too - pony races, waggon races and trotting races. I went there fairly regularly. Thousands of people would turn up. I also went to the pigeon-shooting and I even took part. I won something in '73- a money prize."

Page 142   "Yes, I was there. I remember it well. A silk handkerchief is not much of a prize, but I suppose it's the honour of winning."

"Who knows, she could have got herself in the family way."

Page 144	"Never fear. That's what the tokens are for. Only one train can pass on this stretch of line at a time. It wouldn't happen."

Page 150	"Yes, those were disastrous days. I'll never forget them myself, and you being so ill afterwards.."

Page 158	"Yes, Jane. It was a good day. Thinking of that reminds me of other good times we had. Do you remember the times we went to Cellerhead for the fairs?

Page 159	"Yes, the fairs are mainly for the sale of horses and cattle. They get a good gathering on fair days. But, you're wrong about them not making a living as every Monday these pubs are crowded and the roads packs with farms, butchers, dealers, colliers and all and sundry, coming from far and near to compete in or watch sporting events of all kinds. Of course, there's a lot of booze necked and I've seen a few fights. Remember I took you one Monday and there were wheelbarrow races and such.

Page 160	"Yes, we took the two lads and treated them to rhubarb dipped in sugar. We both had a couple of beers while watching the wrestling."

"Yes, and pigeon shooting. You know I like the shooting, and I had a go. Didn't win anything that day though – the others were too good.

Page 161	Yes, and I won something – some sort of a toy."

"There was a guy doing weight lifting. He claimed to be the strongest man in Staffordshire. He could lift two 90lb weights above his head and knock them together fourteen times! He was introduced as having walked the twenty-one miles to the Cat and Fiddle Inn between Macclesfield and Buxton, for the contest. There was another for Yorkshire – the Yorkshire champion, he was matched against. At one point, the competitors had to pick up a massive stone ball each, run with it, then lift it to place it on top of a 5ft high wall. Our guy won, but it was a close run thing, and for an encore, he lifted up two young ladies, each sitting on an arm, and walked around the paddock with them. He was a massive feller, big and tall with it, with muscles as hard as iron. It was only afterwards, we found out that the Yorkshireman doped our lad's beer to try to turn the match in their favour, but the contest was over before the dope took effect. Then our lad walked the twenty-one miles home."

Page 162   "Of course, you wouldn't remember the bull ring they had there. They stopped it in 1840. It was sat between the Methodist Chapel and the Hope and Anchor Inn, quite near the road. Bull baiting at the time was fairly common then, as a sport. The bull was tethered to an iron ring set in a big stone. Dogs were then slipped in, under the direction of the master of ceremonies, who we called the 'Bellot', and the dogs were set on the bull."

"Yes, you haven't heard the worse. Sometimes, the bull would get loose."
"Yes, he'd run havoc, aggravated as he was, and in pain, charging at everything and everyone that got in his way, even getting out into the main road. I've seen it myself. We'd all had to jump for it

and wait until the bull had come to a stop and calmed down, before the owner could catch it and lead it back to the field.."

Page 163   And talking about cattle, well… cows to be precise. I don't know if you were there the day of the ruckus with Mr Willshaw. It was raining cats and dogs. Anyway, Willshaw bought a cow at Cellarhead, but the man he bought it from had sold it twice. The man who sold it had disappeared by then. They fought for it and the fight went on 'til they could not stand any more. They both got pneumonia and Willshaw died."

"Yes, Jane. I can see that you've been staying up with me all night, in the chair, since you brought me here, and I'm very grateful, but you've not been getting any proper sleep yourself. It's not right, so I'll do my best. I'm feeling a bit better, so I'll give it a try.

Page 166   "Of course, I've slowed down now. I'm getting on and I cannot keep up with the young lads. So I let them do most of the physical hard work, while I've taken over the job of supervisor and planner. I still keep my hand in though."

Page 169   "Yes, William Mellor Meigh was quite different from his father, and probably didn't have the same amount of money, so he used brick, as it was cheaper.

There's someone called George Mountford in there now. He's s in his late 30s and has two men working for him, Charles Heath and William Janes, and he's got his wife, Anne, a young son, George, and his widowed mother-in-law living with him."

Page 170   "Hmm, I believe they had seven children between them and three servents. One ofthem was called Ann Chetwynd, so she must have been related to Dinah Chetwynd, you remember her don't you?"

"Yes, he was an OK kind of man. A bit gruff, but, as long as you did your work, he was fine with you. He's nothing like his father. He can control his temper. You never knew where you were with Job Meigh, up one moment, down the next, with fits of rage. You know yourself, Jane, what he could be like."

Page 171   "Well, he's got a lot to be sorry for, that one, that's all I can say."

"Yes, there's a few ghost stories around this area. A few fellows I know reckon they've seen ghosts. There's supposed to be one under the bridge on the Trent at Harcastle, known as the 'Kidsgrove Boggart'. I've never seen one myself, but I won't say it's fantasy, or strong drink, or the light playing ticks on you as there have been too many people of good character who have seen them, sober, sane people, holding down good jobs.."

Page 173   "Local legend says that, if you run around her grave three times on Halloween, while chanting 'Molly Leigh', Milly Leigh comes out of her grave and chases them away, out of the churchyard.."

"Aw, can't you take a joke? – maybe you are, maybe you're not!"

Page 174   "Job Meigh had a commission agent in '61, living at Mettle House, just below Ash Hall. He was David King and came from Lancashire. He acted as an intermediary in business deals. I believe he sold Job Meigh's pottery ware abroad in return for a share in the profits." I remembered Mettle House as now being the Wise Owl Nursery.

"In 1854 Job Meigh decided to build a pair of labourers' cottages at the corner of Salters Lane, just over the road from Washerwall."

Page 175   "They were in the old sandstone too, like Ash Hall. I was working with William Bonnell, the estate carpenter, and he went to live in one of them in '71, with his family. He moved from Lawson's Farm in Brookhouse Lane. So, he's living there now, with his lady, Sarah, and his son, Charlie, moved out some time ago. He's a coal miner, and his daughter, Annie, is married now. The other cottage is rented by someone called George Sillitoe – he's a gardener and comes from Leek. He was there with his wife and five children. I don't know how they all fitted in as it's only a small cottage. They're a bit of a brood, and two of the girls can't keep a job, I don't know how this George fellow manages. To make matters worse, he also had some woman staying with them, some time ago – she was out of work too."

Page 176   "Yes, I never build like that – it's botched work. I don't know how long they will last."
"In '57 Job Meigh extended the Lodge House by the gate.. In '61 the coachman then was German Dean and his wife, their 5-year-old daughter, and the wife's widower father, who was about 73 then."

Page 177   "So, that's me. What have you been doing yourself, Jane? I know you've got your nursing rounds that keep you busy. Have you got yourself a manfriend? I know you go around with Dr Knight."
"Just asking. You're keeping your age well. I just thought there would be someone."

Page 180   "That will be an improvement, Jane. Looks like it will save lives."

Page 181   About time."

Page 182   "Well, I never."

"You know, I don't think that, Jane."

Page 183   "Yes, I knew all about that when I worked in the potteries before I met you. Terrible – poor mites. But it was the way of live then. Way knew no better, and families had to send their children out to work to earn a living, otherwise they could not earn enough to feed the family." John said, shaking his head.

Page 197   "Ah, we're strong. We can lift anything. We might look puny but we just need feeding up a bit. We've not had anything much in the way of dinners, but we can do it. Just give us a try. We're men now. We've been working since we were 10."

Page 198   "Oh, but that's women's work. We won't do women's work. That's not for the likes of us."

Kevin replied, "Oh, alright. Is there a fancy French name for men doing the washing and such like?"

Page 201   "That's alright, Jane. It's not as if I'm going anywhere fast. No, I'd would like to hear what you've been doing. You've definitely not been sitting on your backside all of these years.."
"Oh, I'm alright. I'm in no pain. Yes, maybe I could do with a bit of exercise – no hills though. I don't know if I'm up for hills."

"That sounds good. It'll get me out of these four walls and I could do with a pint.."

Page 203   "That all sounds very nice, nice warm bath and a good bed, with a doctor to look after you.."

Page 204   "They're not giving me anything proper to eat, because I'm not married, they tell me",
Page 205   "I was broke, starving and ill – could not work. My chest hurts when I coughed and I cough up blood sometimes. They put me on this work – it makes my cough worse. I can't say anything, otherwise they give me a beating."

Page 207   "So, Jane, it looks like things have got worse since you were working there in '71?"

Page 210   "They're almost free of it – it must have been something they've eaten or dirt, or a bit of the two."

If there are knives and such or medicines, it's because I get them out. I have to buy them out of my own pay and I get just £20 a year. So they get what they get.

Page 211   "So, the infirmary was in a right state. God help them."
"Oh, you must not go in there."

"There's someone comes in every so often to see to the patients in there. See, they've got smallpox. She's another inmate like me, but she's had smallpox herself, so the Master has got her in to treat them."

"If you insist, miss." and she duly opened the door for me.

Page 212   "I don't know, Mrs. There's a woman who comes every so often to feed us and clean us and I've seen the door open, with a man looking in, but that is all, and we haven't seen the woman for some time. We're ever so hungry. I don't know if Peter here is alive. I cannot seem to wake him."

Page 213   "Oh, but I need it, miss. Don't take my drink away from me.."

Page 216   "Poppycock. 'How did they reach their positions. Seems like they could not organise a piss-up in a brewery." Replied John, "One side did not know what the other side was doing, with the guardians appointing who they wanted, not caring about suitability or experience, plus the LGB war epected to approve such appointments without question!"

"They're not all bad though, surely? There's gott to be some good ones?

"Does he just attend, or is he medicating the patients?"

Page 219   Well, it fare well bothers me and I'm right scared. I've also seen weird lights, green and orange lights coming from the room a couple of times. I told Dinah about it and we both got our courage up to peak round the door ….. well I don't want to be someone who makes a lot of fuss but I'm really bothered and all of a fluster."

"Well, Dinah told me to come tell you… but, well, and I'm all a tremble, after what we've seen."

".. Well, the room was freezing. I could seen my breathe. We looked round the door and there was this light, sort of shimmering orange and green. We couldn't make it out at first, but then it took a sort of shape – that of a young lad…. I think, ma'm, we've seen a ghost."

Page 226   "Yes, it was a bit of a squeeze with that crowd, I couldn't go anywhere, so I had to put up with you."

"Well, I couldn't see you being pushed and shoved in the crowd. So, I stayed.

Page 227   "If you say so, and I thought I was safe – you couldn't put a spell on me on church grounds."

Yes, people wanted something bigger and more elegant, and a considerable amount of money was obtained from Lichfield Diocesan Church Society and Incorporated Society, as well as parish rates and private subscriptions."

Page 228   "In the meantime, work commenced on demolishing the old building. As you said, the old church was ancient. I believe they tried to rebuild it in 1716 from stones taking from Hulton Abbey. The chancel arch and chancel itself were brought over, the the abbey, although at different times."

"The new church was to be built about fifty yards to the south of the old one, on a bit higher ground and be an attractive addition to the village generally, with the spire being a striking crown to the whole edifice. I managed to have a look at the plans beforehand. They wanted a nave about 60ft long, with a south aisle about the same length."

Page 229   "Yes, I remember it being a bit windy, but luckily it didn't rain. We were standing there for ages, listening to him. He's a good man, but a long windbag, that's for sure."

Page 230   "True, I suppose, and it was a good, religious speech, suitable for the evet, and everyone was listening intently."
"Alright, come on, if you must, I know you're dying to."

Page 234   "No, it's too much like a courtroom. Do you know, they hold prisoners there, in that little cottage over the road, opposite? There's an underground tunnel leading to the pub – they bring prisoners through the tunnel to the pub for their hearing with the magistrate."

Pagae 235 "Yes, Job Meigh didn't look too happy, especially as he was on the building committee, and his son, William was elected Chairman. Did you know too, that Job Meigh had donated £100 towards the building costs aside from advancing money to pay the builder during the course of the construction? Mind you – it was a great service – a blessing on the church. Come to think of it, no, they had to get an Anglican and Job Meigh was still a prominent member of the Bethesda Methodist New Connexion Chapel, at this time, in Hanley, so he wouldn't be up for it.

Page 236 "Yes, I saw the obituary that appeared in the Staffordshire Sentinel. I went along to see the hearse, but stood outside, didn't go in."

Page 240 "She could have been sick. It was not long after that, about a year, that she herself died."

"Yes, he was not a nice man."

Page 241 "Yes, talking about funerals, do you remember the funeral of Hugh Bourne? It was in '52. He'd lived at Fort Hayes Farm, just right off Clough Road. He was a Primitive Methodist, following Wesleyan methods, and used to preach in the open air. He was well loved around here. They even accepted women preachers, what about that! Anyway, he died on 11th October 1852 and his funeral was attended by 16,000 people!"

Page 245   "Oh, that's a sad story."
"Yes, but I'm not a forgiving sort. If I'm hurt, I'm hurt for a long time. It's a sort of self-protection.."

"OK, you've got my attention."

Page 247   "Yes, I've heard that story before. My nephew, Charlie, from Tunstall, told it to me. So poignant and moving."

"I don't know, but I'll give it a try."

Page 248   "That's two things, you're not giving me a chance."
"Right, you know I like my railway history – from 1864 Stoke houses the repair shops of the North Staffordshire Railway and Kerr Stuart & Co Ltd, the independent railway locomotive manufacturers had taken up residence there, just this year. Basically, all of Britain is covered by railroads now. We can import and export to all over the world."
"I've got something else, as you had two goes. In 1870, a borough fire brigade was established, at last, although the brigade was required to act as special constables, when necessary. I told you that as we were going round Etruria to see the official 'cutting of the sod' ceremony, taking place in a field, for the new railway – remember when the man broke his silver spade."

Page 249   "Yes, this meant that the Trent and Mersey Canal, built 60 years earlier, lost all of its trade. Clay could be imported much quicker by rail. And, of course, the six towns started to grow with more people coming in. Burslem, the mother town, was still largest though."

"In the 1840s Elias Howe was the first American to invent a sewing machine. Also, this decade saw the invention of the first vulcanised rubber pneumatic tyre, the first gain elevator, and the first stapler."

Page 250   "In 1845, the new town hall was opened in Fountain Square and the police station moved there."

In 1847 The Hanley County Court District was established – it originally covered the whole of the Potteries with the court meeting at Hanley Town Hall."

"So, further away, in 181 there was the Great Exhibition at Crystal Palace. Yes, it was constructed from a cast iron frame and glass. I heard that six million people attended – about 1/3r of the entire population of Great Britain! It also featured the first public conveniences, each person paying 1 penny to use them."

Page 251   "That's nothing. Elisha Otis invented the lift. I've never seen one in operation and I think I might be a bit scared to go into one, but they say he builds in an automatic spring-operated brake system to stop the cab from falling if the cable were to break.."

"Wake up. Are you daydreaming?" I heard John say. "It's your turn."
Page 252   "In 1855 they built the Panama Railway crossing from the Atlantic all the way over to the Pacific. This led onto the

building of the Panama Canal itself. They couldn't have one without the other."

"Ay, I'm not having that. You said from 1842. That's before that time."

"Alright, I've got another. The Pullman train sleeping car, names after its inventor, George Pullman."

Page 253 "Henry Bessemer developed his converter in 1857. Previously steel had been too expensive to produce, and was only used in small, expensive items, such as knives, swords and armour.

Page 254 "1859 saw William Smith drilling 60ft down and discovering oil in Pennsylvania. They're getting out about 20 barrels a day now. This was the first oil taken from underground. Before that, they cod only collect oil that had bubbled to the surface into pools. No-one knew what they had at first – they were drilling for water found oil and closed the well down. Silly sods."

"Let's get away from America. London installed its first underground railway, 'The Metropolitan Railway', between Paddington Station and Farringdon Street via King's Cross.

Page 255 The bronze statue of Josiah Wedgewood, opposite the railway station, was erected in 1863 and the next year saw the opening of the Stoke railway works of the North Staffordshire Railway. Oh, and also, Stoke City Football Club was founded around the same time. The team was now big enough to have a football club, and all because of the railways coming.

311

I know I said I didn't want anything about America, but I suppose it counts. The Civil War ended in 1865 and then, on the 14th April, President Lincoln was shot and mortally wounded by John Wilks Booth, while at the theatre."

"I believe, in the same year, Alfred Nobel invented dynamite."
Page 256   "During the American Civil War in the 1860s, Richard Gatling patented his machine gun, named after him, and Robert Whitehead invented the torpedo. George Westinghouse also invented air brakes, and tungsten steel was first made."

Page 257   "No, we're always at the end of the queue!"
"And getting back to football – Port Vale Football Club was established in 1876."

"I think it was a tie, myself, so how about we do the two?"

Page 261   "I don't know anything about this. I don't believe you. It makes no sense. I didn't die down a mine shaft. I'm still here, which you can see for yourself."

"Yes, I remember all of that. I'd realised I loved her. She was dying and she was calling out, that she wanted to stay. I didn't understand it at the time, but I suppose I do now. She wanted to be with me and didn't want to return to the 21st century."

Page 263   "Can you forgive me, Jane? I've been ignorant all this time, but I see now that I was wrong. Can we make amends? Is it too late? I've never stopped loving you."

So, what do you think, Alfred? Your ma and pa are getting back together."

Page 269   'He may not have suffered. Hold onto that thought. We know your spirit was with him to the end. Anyhow, we know he's save now."

"Jane was looking after him. Shey wouldn't have let him suffer. Think about that, love."

Acknowledgements
www.thepotteries.org
The language of the Potteries
North Staffordshire Dialect – Vowel pronunciation guide
Lillydale colliery Explosion 1881 – researched by John Lumsdon
Mervyn Edwards – Historian
Sheffield Telegraph
Ancestry.com
Spartacus Educational
Wetherspoon News Spring 2019
Staffordshire Advertiser 22 April 1854
Staffordshire Advertiser 29 June 1881
Bucknall – a Hole Wears Longer than a Patch – Elizabeth W Bass
From Wetley Moor to Bucknall Sands by Elizabeth W Bass
Werrington – Yesterday's Voice by Elizabeth W Bass
Werrington – Some Notes on its History by J D Johnstone
Notes on Nursing by Florence Nightingale
North Staffordshire Medical Institute 1965
When I was a Child – autobiography of Charles Shaw
National Archives
Everyday Life in 19th Century Britain – by Tim Lambert
Libcom.org
Google searches